# BOOST YOUR DEFENCE TO FIGHT DISEASES

DR. JAGATJIT SINGH VIRK

# Dedication

To my wife and kids Pushwaz & Parwaz for their love and support

# TABLE OF CONTENTS


What is Immunity? ...............................................................1
Types of Immunity ..............................................................2
Signs and symptoms of weakened Immunity .........................14
Diet ................................................................................15
Exercise ..........................................................................17
Sleep ..............................................................................20
Stress..............................................................................25
Vitamin A ........................................................................29
Vitamin B ........................................................................31
Vitamin C ........................................................................32
Vitamin D ........................................................................36
Vitamin E.........................................................................39
Obesity............................................................................44
Iodine .............................................................................48
Fasting ............................................................................55
Sauna ..............................................................................57
Deep Breathing .................................................................59
Magnesium .......................................................................63
Cancer.............................................................................66
Autoimmunity....................................................................72
Positive Attitude ................................................................80
Gratitude ..........................................................................83
Gut Immunology..................................................................87
Strategies to boost immunity ..................................................91
(a) Turmeric (The golden spice)..............................................98
(b) Cinnamon (Cinnamomum zeylanicum) ...............................101
(c) Black Cumin Seed (Nigella sativa)....................................103
(d) Neem (Azadirachta indica) .............................................105
(e) Garlic (Allium sativum) .................................................108
(f) Onion (Allium cepa)......................................................111
(g) Ginger (Zingiber officinale)............................................114
Definitions and Key concepts...............................................118
What we should know about COVID-19 ...................................124

# INTRODUCTION

Today is my first day of writing my new book on a topic that is very close to my heart. I have been practicing medicine for fifty years and taken care of thousands of patients. I am using this opportunity to write this book to share my experience about preventing disease by boosting our immunity. My goal is to provide basic education to the public about how to improve their health and eliminate or control diseases with routine life-style changes, natural and easy to practice methods. The focus will be mostly on common diseases but I have also discussed some rare conditions. I will also give diverse types of diet plans and exercises to improve our health. One thing we must understand that it is not the doctor or medicine which cures us but our own body which cures us from ailments. Doctors and medicines only provide support to our body. Take example of AIDS patients, who have been robbed of their immune system and any infection which may be trivial for a normal healthy person can prove to be deadly to these patients because their body can't protect itself.

Another example is of a repair of a building. We supply the instructions and drawing plans to the builder and ask the builder to construct or repair the building which they do to our specifications. The same type of builder is within our being, which builds and repairs the building, our body in a comparable way. We must supply the raw material for that process to occur to our body in the form of diet and nutrition just as we provide the builder construction material in the form of bricks, cement sand and wood and steel.

Currently, our immunity is even more important due to the COVID-19 pandemic which has created panic in the society. The scientifically proven precautions are to use three-layered masks, keeping a distance of six feet between two individuals and washing hands with soap and water for more than twenty seconds or using a reliable sanitizer. Nature has also given us at least six protective layers on our face in the form of 1, Skin for our mechanical protection. 2. Sebum containing free fatty acids to fight the bugs. 3. Hair or cilia in our nose. 4. Mucus to trap the microorganisms, 5. The IgA antibody secreted in the lining and is, for our protection locally. 6. Normal micro biota of our orifices which protect us from the pathogenic bugs. These are the natural forces of nature which protect us from the onslaught of external invaders on our body. The only precaution we can take is to keep it optimally healthy with proper, natural, fresh and organic nutrients. This should be in addition to keeping our body fully fit with proper exercise including stretching, strengthening, aerobic and balancing exercises.

Complementary medicine is growing in popularity. A future without drugs will probably never materialize, but people are waking up to the idea that tools to help prevent and cure illnesses without drugs are at our disposal right now. We can't cure all illnesses without medical intervention, of course, but we can influence one of the problems of the modern life-style: The- disconnect with our bodies and environment.

Your mental state influences your physical health. There is irrefutable evidence to show that positive thinking can make you healthier. When one examines how the body works, it's easy to see. The functions of the brain are more chemical reactions. Synapses fire when we make thoughts, and our immune and lymphatic systems are chemical based. We are essentially a collection of chemicals, from our brains to our bones.

We cannot fulfill our daily needs of nutrients by taking our normal diet alone. We have to supplement it with adequate supplements. For example, our required daily intake of Vitamin C is only 60 mg per day to prevent scurvy, but a large dose of Vitamin C is required to protect us from myocardial damage and stroke. Similarly, the dose required for Co Q 10 cannot be fulfilled only from the diet which will require eating large amount of fat, which may prove to be deleterious to the body. Moreover, our diet lacks essential nutrients as compared to the fifty years ago, because of poor content of nutrients in soil due to depletion, usage of chemical fertilizers and pesticides as well as calorie dense diet which reduce the total amount of fiber and food content that we eat. So, it is vital to ensure that our diet is perfect in all respects.

# PREFACE

This book is written to help boost the morale of my patients and public in this pandemic of COVID-19. I have tried to inform the public through this book that you and only you can defend your body against any attack of the external micro-organisms with your changed behavior and correcting your life-style. God has given us every weapon to fight the disease, but we have forgotten the blessing of nature in this materialistic journey of life and discarded the simple and natural ways of leading our lives. By trapping ourselves in the allure of industrialized world, we have inculcated bad habits leading to life-style and chronic diseases like coronary artery disease, obesity, diabetes, respiratory illnesses, neuro-psychiatric and auto-immune conditions etc. Our innate resistance to fight these maladies has been seriously compromised. We can change this by reverting to natural ways of living. I hope that this book will guide you to change a few of your habits creating a silver lining in this COVID-19 pandemic and leading to a healthy and fulfilling life now and beyond!

Dr Jagatjit Singh Virk

November 27, 2020

# CHAPTER 1

## What is Immunity?

"The Doctors of the future will give no medicine but will instruct his patients in care of the human frame, in diet, and in the cause and prevention of disease."        -Thomas Edison


Immunity is the capability of the living being to resist the harmful microorganisms and toxins which attack the body. The quality or state of being immune is achieved by preventing the actions of microorganisms, or by counteracting the effects of their products. The microorganisms may be bacteria, viruses, or fungi, or their toxins. Immunity can be defined as a complex biological system with the ability to recognize and tolerate whatever belongs to itself, and to recognize and reject what is foreign (non-self).

# CHAPTER 2

## Types of Immunity

"Human body has been designed to resist an infinite number of changes and attacks brought about by its environment. The secret of good health lies in successful adjustment to changing stresses on the body." – Harry J. Johnson

There are four types of immunity in the human body:

- ACTIVE immunity: The body makes its own antibodies to protect itself from external threats of microorganisms and toxins.

- PASSIVE immunity: The body gets antibodies from the external source like an infant gets antibodies from her mother and from the anti-venom vaccine to the patient.

- NATURAL immunity: There is not any deliberate contact with the patient but the person gets the natural immunity from the environment, just like herd immunity.

- ARTIFICIAL immunity: The short acting immunity is gained through blood transfusion of mono-clonal antibodies.

The immune system consists of a team of cells, proteins, tissues and organs. The children do not have fully developed immune system. That is the reason children have more infections in the childhood and less in the adulthood.

There are two main diseases of the immune system, these are

1) Primary immune deficiency syndrome, where the immunity is primarily deficient from birth and

2)   2) Secondary or the Acquired immune deficiency syndrome where the disease is acquired in the later life. In both the cases, body's ability to cope up with the external aggression of microorganism is compromised and any opportunistic infection can over- powers the body and makes it sick.

The primary lymphoid organs are the bone marrow and thymus. They create special immune cells called **Lymphocytes**. The secondary lymphoid organs include lymph glands, spleen, tonsils, and certain tissues in the mucus membrane layers of the body, just as in the Peyer's patches of gastrointestinal tract.

The immune system works in five ways:

## THE INNATE SYSTEM

This system is the general system of immunity where it is effective against all types of foreign invaders. Moreover, this is our first line of defense against these intruders in our body. This system consists of our skin, mucus membrane, cilia and hair, mucus, friendly flora on our body, saliva and tears, and free fatty acid layer secreted by our apocrine glands. This system traps the invader at the point of entry and destroys it there and then. The surface immune globulin A (S IgA) may be included in this which works here. Mucus is designed to trap offending viruses, which are efficiently and quickly expelled from the body through coughing and sneezing. Fever—Fevers fight influenza viruses. Because viruses are sensitive to temperature changes and cannot survive above normal body heat, your body uses fever to help destroy them.

## THE INTERFERON SYSTEM

This system is especially important against the viruses. Virus infected cells produce and release small proteins called interferon, which play a role in immune protection against viruses. These prevent replication of viruses by directly interfering with their ability to replicate within an infected cell. Interferon, or IFNs, is proteins that are made and released in response to pathogens like viruses, bacteria, parasites, and cancer cells. Interferon plays a key role as the first line of defense against infections. IFNs are part of the non-specific immune system.

There are **three types of interferon** (**IFN**), 1) alpha, 2) beta and 3) gamma. IFN-alpha is produced in the leukocytes infected with virus, while IFN-beta is from fibroblasts infected with virus. IFN-gamma is induced by the stimulation of sensitized lymphocytes with antigen or non-sensitized lymphocytes with mitogens.

**Licorice** increases production of interferon, the body's natural antiviral compound. It blocks viruses, and activates macrophage and natural killer cell activity, helping to get your immune system working. And it has antibiotic activity against staph, strep, and Candida, among others.

## THE ADAPTIVE SYSTEM

This system is specific for a particular invader and is sometimes called a humoral immunity. Lymphocytes from the bone marrow called B cells are the major contributor to this system. B cells produce specific types of antibodies, which target the specific microorganisms. Antibodies lock into the antigen of the organism, but they do not kill it, only mark it for death. The killing is the job of other cells, such as phagocytes like neutrophils and macrophages.

Specific immunity is characterized by greater specificity and less speed than the natural immune response. Lymphocytes have receptor sites on their cell surfaces. The receptor on each cell fits with one and only one small molecular shape, or antigen, on a given invader and therefore responds to one and only one kind of invader. When activated, these antigen-specific cells divide to create a population of cells with the same antigen specificity in a process called *clonal proliferation,* or the *proliferative response.* Although this process is efficient in terms of the number of cells that must be supported on a day-to-day basis, it creates a delay of up to several days before a full defense is mounted, and the body must rely on natural immunity to contain the infection during this time.

There are three types of lymphocytes that mediate specific immunity: T-helper cells, T-Cytotoxic cells, and B cells. The main function of **T-helper** cells is to produce cytokines that direct and amplify the rest of the immune response. **T-Cytotoxic** cells recognize antigen expressed by cells that are infected with viruses or otherwise compromised (e.g., cancer cells) and lyses those cells. **B cells** produce soluble proteins called *antibody* that can perform several functions, including neutralizing bacterial toxins, binding to free virus to prevent its entry into cells, and opsonization, in which a coating of antibody increases the effectiveness of natural immunity.

Antibodies are a large family of chemicals called immunoglobulin, which play many roles in the immune system. These are of several types:

- Immunoglobulin G (IgG): It marks the microbes and other cells can recognize and deal with them.

- Immunoglobulin M (IgM): This is expert in killing bacteria and is a large molecule that clears antigen from the bloodstream.

- Immunoglobulin A (IgA): It congregates in fluids, such as tears and saliva, where it protects the gateways into the body.

- Immunoglobulin E (IgE): It protects against the parasites and is also to blame for allergy.

- Immunoglobulin D (IgD): It stays bound to B lymphocytes helping them to start the immune response.

An important immunological development is the recognition that specific immunity in humans is composed of cellular and humoral responses. Cellular immune responses are mounted against intracellular pathogens like viruses and are coordinated by a subset of T-helper lymphocytes called **Th1 cells**. In the Th1 response, the T-helper cell produces cytokines, including IL-2 and interferon gamma (IFN γ). These cytokines selectively activate T-Cytotoxic cells as well as natural killer cells. Humoral immune responses are mounted against extracellular pathogens such as parasites and bacteria; they are coordinated by a subset of T-helper lymphocytes called **Th2 cells**. In the Th2 response, the T-helper cell produces different cytokines, including IL-4 and IL-10, which selectively activate B cells and mast cells to combat extracellular pathogens.

## THE MICRO BIOME SYSTEM

Micro biome consists of 60 trillion bacteria i.e. ten times of our bodily cells, 360 trillions of viruses and many more other microorganisms on our body. All together, they contain 99% of the total genome in the body. That is the reason these microbes have a key role in our life. 70 to 80 percent of our immunity lies in our gut due to the presence of this micro biota.

The micro biota plays a fundamental role on the induction, training, and function of the host immune system. In return, the immune system has largely evolved to maintain the symbiotic relationship of the host with these highly diverse and evolving microbes. When operating optimally this immune system–micro biota alliance allows the induction of protective responses to pathogens and the maintenance of regulatory pathways involved in the maintenance of tolerance to innocuous antigens. However, in high-income countries overuse of antibiotics, changes in diet, and elimination of constitutive partners such as nematodes has selected for a micro biota that lack the resilience and diversity needed to establish balanced immune responses. This phenomenon is proposed to account for some of the dramatic rise in autoimmune and inflammatory disorders in parts of the world where our symbiotic relationship with the micro biota has been the most affected.

The immune system is composed of a complex network of innate and adaptive components endowed with an extraordinary ability to adapt and respond to highly diverse challenges. Collectively this cellular network acts as a formidable regulator of host homeostasis allowing sustaining and restoring tissue function in the context of microbial and environmental encounters. The development of defined arms of the immune system and more particularly the ones associated with adaptive immunity has coincided with the acquisition of a complex micro biota supporting the concept that a large fraction of this machinery has evolved as a means to maintain a symbiotic relationship with these highly diverse microbial communities. In turn the micro biota promotes and calibrates all aspects of the immune system.

When running optimally, the immune system - micro biota alliance interweaves the innate and adaptive arms of immunity in a dialogue that selects, calibrates and terminates responses in the most appropriate manner. However, both the acquisition of a complex immune system and its reliance on the micro biota came at a price. Pathologies that increasingly affect humans such as allergies, autoimmune and inflammatory disorders all arise from a failure to control misdirected immune responses against self, micro biota derived or environmental antigens. Further, alteration of the composition and function of the micro biota because of antibiotic use, diet evolution and recent elimination of constitutive partners such as helminthes worms has transformed our microbial allies into potential liabilities. Although members of the micro biota are often referred to as commensally the symbiosis - persistent interaction- between the micro biota and its mammalian host encompasses various forms of relationship including mutuality, parasitic or commensally. However, how defined members of the micro biota interact with their host can be highly contextual with the same microbe developing as mutualism or parasite according to the nutritional, co-infection or genetic landscape of its host. Over the past decade, exploration of optimal and deregulated partnerships between the micro biota and its mammalian host has taken center stage in the field of immunology and led to the re-discovery of a more holistic view of host physiology. Indeed, the notion that microbial partners can promote human health is not a recent concept and was originally proposed by the seminal work of Döderlein (1892) and his understanding of the role of lactobacilli as gatekeepers of the vaginal ecosystem as well as the observation of Metchnikoff associating prolonged life with fermented milk products. Recent sequencing efforts of the human meta-genome have changed our understanding of the micro biome and how variations in these populations can contribute to disease states.

A large fraction of the immune system's function is aimed at controlling our relationship with the micro biota. As such the highest number of immune cells in the body is resident at sites colonized by commensals such as the skin or the GI tract. In order to protect their ecological niche, a dominant action of the healthy micro biota on the immune system is aimed at reinforcing barrier immunity and therefore their own containment. A central strategy used by the host to maintain its homeostatic relationship with the micro biota is to minimize contact between microorganisms and the epithelial cell surface thereby limiting tissue inflammation and microbial translocation. In the gastrointestinal tract, home to the largest density of commensals, this segregation is carried out by the combined action of epithelial cells, mucus, IgA, antimicrobial peptides and immune cells. Collectively these structural and immunological components have been referred to as the "mucosal firewall"

Tissues that are natural habitats of the micro biota such as the skin, the GI tract or the lungs are also the portals by which pathogens access the host and often the primary site of infections. This implies that the first encounter of pathogens with the immune system occurs in an environment conditioned and regulated by its endogenous micro biota. As such the fate of commensals and pathogens (as well as their classification) is highly interdependent. Notably, commensals can directly and dynamically interact with pathogens and immune cells and the results of this interaction can define the pathogenesis and outcome of a given infection.

The protective effect of the micro biota has been revealed in clinical and experimental settings in which broad antibiotic treatment can allow the domination of intestinal micro biota with drug resistant microbes such as vancomycin resistant enterococcus (VRE), a pathogen that causes bloodstream infections in immune-compromised patients. Infections caused by multidrug-resistant organisms are on the rise and have developed into endemic and epidemic situations worldwide. Harnessing the micro biota to combat these infections represents an important therapeutic avenue with the most spectacular results obtained thus far in the context of *Clostridium difficile* colitis (Fecal Transplantation). During this recurrent infection, transfer of a micro biota from a healthy donor eradicated the infection with a remarkable efficiency. Again highlighting the concept of defined microbes endowed with superior adjuvant capacity, the protective effect of the micro biota in VRE infected patient was highly dependent on the presence of the commensal *Barnesiella*.

The skin, the largest organ of the body, is a critical interface between the host and the environment. Unbiased microbial sequencing has shown the presence of highly diverse and specific commensal niches along distinct topographical sites of the skin. Although the skin is a rather inhospitable environment, poor in nutrients and moisture, up to 1 billion bacteria inhabit a typical square centimeter of human skin, covering the surface and extending down into the sebaceous glands and hair follicles. In contrast to the known role of the gut micro biota in promoting the gastrointestinal associated lymphoid tissue (GALT) development, skin commensals are not required for the development of associated lymphoid tissue. The skin resident bacteria, such as *Staphylococcus epidermidis,* can control fundamental aspects of local immunity and tissue repair. Skin commensals do not affect the capacity of T cells to be primed or to migrate to the skin but modulate dermal T cell function by tuning the cutaneous inflammatory milieu and more particularly the production of IL-1α that in turn directly controls the capacity of dermal resident T cells to produce inflammatory cytokines such as IFN-γ and IL-17A. Thus, in contrast to the role of the gut micro biota, the action of skin commensals on the local immune system is discrete and highly compartmentalized.

The oral cavity also harbors a unique and complex microbial community accumulating on both the hard and soft oral tissues in sessile bio-films. One of the proposed roles of the oral micro biome on the immune system is associated with its capacity to promote inflammasome activity leading to the local increase of the inflammatory cytokine IL1β. At other sites such as the lung or vaginal mucosa the role of commensals on tissue immunity remains largely unknown. In the absence of commensals, the number of infiltrating Th2 lymphocytes and eosinophils was elevated and the composition and status of activation of lung dendritic cells was altered during airway inflammation. Immune system is our savior of all foreign attacks of microorganisms on our body and we should leave no stone unturned to keep it perfectly fit and fine to combat these invaders. Sometimes with our wrong habits we do not care to keep this system optimal and at that time, we succumb to the onslaught of these foreign intruders and lose the battle.

## NEURAL SYSTEM

Neural system of the body is mainly governed by our brain and central nervous system (nerves) and is separated from the body's immune system by the blood-brain barrier. However, the central nervous system has its own immune system called the 'neuro-immune' system that protects it from infection and foreign cells. Alterations in the state and function of the nervous system influence the immune response. The nervous system regulates innate immune responses through the release of neurotransmitters, neuro-peptides and neuro-hormones. The Vagus nerve, the tenth cranial nerve, has direct connection with the brain and is a major part of **Gut-Brain Axis**.

Important insights into the neural control of inflammation have come from the study of a prototypical example of a neural immune-regulatory circuit termed the "inflammatory reflex." In this reflex, afferent signals transmitted through the Vagus nerve are processed in the CNS and culminate in efferent Vagus nerve activity that regulates macrophage cytokine release in the spleen. Our current understanding of this reflex is based on several seminal discoveries. Watkins et al. and other research teams found that the fever response to low doses of IL-1β injected into the intra-peritoneal cavity of rats requires an intact Vagus nerve, because animals with a sub-diaphragmatically severed Vagus nerve failed to develop a fever response to the injected cytokine. Moreover, injection of IL-1β into the portal vein in rats gives rise to increased afferent activity in the Vagus nerve and increased activity in the splenic nerve, but not when the hepatic branch of the Vagus nerve had been ablated. Thus, signaling in the Vagus nerve plays a role in the systemic response to cytokines.

The parasympathetic state reduces inflammation in your body. It is the vagus nerve that serves as a detection system for inflammation. The vagus nerve's vast network of fibers stationed around the organs identify inflammation (such as the presence of inflammatory proteins) and alert your brain to send out anti- inflammatory signals, in essence helping to prevent chronic inflammation in your body.

Chronic or excessive inflammation can be linked to heart disease, auto-immunity, and loss of cognitive abilities and often results when we are unable to drop into the parasympathetic state.

The parasympathetic state helps improve communication between your body and your brain to help modulate your inflammatory response. In the parasympathetic state, your vagus nerve communicates with the rest of the body by releasing the neuro-transmitter acetyl-choline which acts as a brake on inflammation in your body, inhibiting the production of pro-inflammatory messengers. The ability of your vagus nerve to send signals to your body can be compromised from chronic stress and toxins like heavy metals. To ensure optimal vagal signaling, apply the Parasympathetic enhancing protocols for proper functioning.

Research has shown strong decrease in inflammatory symptoms from stimulating the Parasympathetic state and vagus nerve stimulation seems to restore the body's natural balance. It reduces the over-production of the chemicals messengers that causes chronic inflammation but does not affect healthy immune function, so the body can respond normally to infection.

The parasympathetic state turns on your IMMUNE processes, allowing your body to fight pathogens, bacteria, fungus, parasites, viruses and infections. The sympathetic "fight and flight" state depresses immune function, opening the door to pathogens and chronic infections. This can create a vicious cycle as chronic infections put you into an inflamed state which further triggers the sympathetic nervous system.

More specifically, dysbiotic conditions, like yeast, fungus, and bacterial overgrowth, SIBO, or parasitic infestations all profoundly affect your capacity to absorb nutrients. Later inflammation and toxicity disrupt all of your homeostatic systems of digestion.

The Para-sympathetic state affects EVERY aspect of your well-being!

Digestion, detoxification, and immune function are only turned on when your body is in a parasympathetic state. You should optimally be in a parasympathetic state 80% of the time, but many people struggle to be in this state at any point during their day. This is because stress inhibits the parasympathetic response and the body's essential healing processes shut down.

Consider Parasympathetic state for chronic infections like:

- H Pylori

- Candida

- Fungal infections

- Periodontal infections (Parasympathetic state triggers saliva in mouth)

- Chronic sinus, Respiratory, Gut, or Urinary infections

When the vagus nerve is compromised, you cannot drop into the parasympathetic state and heal. Two things compromise the vagus nerve:

1. Toxic thoughts or stress

2. Physical toxins, infections, or viruses

There are many ways to strengthen the vagus nerve like gargling, singing, chanting, humming, stroking the throat, Probiotics use, meditation, omega 3 fatty acid use, exercise, and massaging.

There are potential signs and symptoms of damaged vagus nerve, which include:

- Loss of gag reflex

- Voice which is hoarse and wheezy

- Trouble drinking liquids

- Difficulty speaking or loss of voice

- Pain in the ear

- Unusual heart rate

- Abnormal blood pressure

- Decreased production of stomach acid

Research shows that **Limonene** found in limes is known to stimulate the production of glutathione (a master anti-oxidant), which helps regulate your immune system probably through parasympathetic route. Unfortunately, most nutritional supplements of glutathione are not absorbed well and do not raise glutathione levels within the cells, so limes ability to help stimulate the production of glutathione inside your cells contributes to the support of immune function.

# CHAPTER 3

## Signs and symptoms of weakened Immunity

"Health is a state of complete harmony of the body, mind and spirit. When one is free from physical disabilities and mental distractions, the gates of the soul open." – B.K.S. Iyenger

A few signs and symptoms of the weakened immune system include:

- We feel tired, all the time.

- Our stress level is quite high.

- We always have a cold.

- We have lots of stomach problems.

- Our wounds are slow to heal.

- We have frequent infections.

These are a few of the signs of the weakened immune system and in this pandemic of COVID 19; we all should try to boost the immunity to optimal levels so that we do not succumb to the foreign invaders.

# CHAPTER 4

# Diet

"To ensure good health: eat lightly, breathe deeply, live moderately, cultivate cheerfulness, and maintain an interest in life." – William Londen

Like any fighting force, the immune system army marches when it's well fed. Healthy immune system warriors need good, regular nourishment. Scientist has long recognized that people who live in poverty and are malnourished are more vulnerable to infectious diseases.

There is evidence that various micronutrient deficiencies- for example, deficiencies of zinc, selenium, iron, copper, folic acid, and vitamins A, B6, C, and E alter immune responses in animals. So, what can you do to improve your immune system? If you suspect your diet is not providing you with all your micronutrient needs- maybe, for instance, if you don't like vegetables, taking a daily multi-vitamin and mineral supplement may bring other health benefits, beyond any possibly beneficial effects on the immune system.

Inter dependence of diet, immune system, and micro-biota interactions are particularly important. Evidence now exists for bi-directional communication between the three key factors in the gastrointestinal track: diet, immune system, and commensal micro flora. Diet can have profound influence on the immune system (e.g. Vitamin A, Vitamin D, iron, folates and AHR ligands), while the immune system can also affect dietary intake through its absorption and assimilation. Diet also has dominant influence on the composition and metabolic capacity of commensal bacteria. While this in return, influence nutrient absorption and fermentation. The immune system can exert control over both commensal composition and localization through metabolites, short chain fatty acids, nutrients and TLR/NO ligands, while commensal signals are critical for development and function of the immune system, through IgA, AMPS, Reg III $\gamma$, Nitric oxide, and Reactive Oxygen Species.

# CHAPTER 5

# Exercise

"Physical fitness is the first requisite of happiness." – Joseph Pilates

During and after physical exercise, pro- and anti-inflammatory cytokines are released, lymphocyte circulation increases, as well as cell recruitment. Such practice has an effect on the lower incidence, intensity of symptoms and mortality in viral infections observed in people who practice physical activity regularly, and its correct execution must be considered to avoid damage. The initial response is given mainly by type I interferon (IFN-I), which drive the action macrophages and lymphocytes, followed by lymphocyte action. A suppression of the IFN-I response has been noted in COVID-19. Severe conditions have been associated with storms of pro-inflammatory cytokines and lymphopenia, as well as circulatory changes and virus dispersion to other organs. The practice of physical activities strengthens the immune system, suggesting a benefit in the response to viral communicable diseases. Thus, regular practice of adequate intensity is suggested as an auxiliary tool in strengthening and preparing the immune system for diseases.

As discussed earlier, the immune response is made of two stages, **innate immunity** and **Adaptive immunity**. The first stage, includes physical and chemical barriers and the action of cells such as macrophages, dendritic cells (DCs), natural killer cells (NK), neutrophils and molecules such as cytokines, interleukins (ILs), nitric oxide (NO) and superoxide anion ($O_2-$). The second one has as mechanism of action the T lymphocytes (TCD4 + and TCD8 +)

and B lymphocytes and their products, such as antibodies and cytokines. Furthermore, the adaptive immune response can be subdivided into cellular immunity (mediated by cells as macrophages and lymphocytes) and humoral immunity (mediated by antibodies). The regular practice of physical exercises promotes improvements in quality of life and can act in the immune response, reducing the risk of developing systemic inflammatory processes and stimulating cellular immunity.

Physical activity is considered one of the vital ingredients of healthy living. In addition to the functions related to the prevention of excess body weight, systemic inflammation and chronic non-communicable diseases, a potential benefit of physical exercise in reducing communicable diseases, including viral pathologies, has been proven by research.

The practice of physical exercise, both in its acute form and in its chronic form, significantly alters the immune system. Studies show that the modulation of the immune response related to exercise depends on factors such as regularity, intensity, duration and type of effort applied.

Moderate-intensity physical exercises stimulate cellular immunity, while prolonged or high-intensity practices without proper rest can trigger decreased cellular immunity, increasing the propensity for infectious diseases. According to the International Society for Exercise and Immunology (ISEI), the immunological decrease occurs after the practice of prolonged physical exercise, that is, after 90 min of moderate- to high-intensity physical activity.

The benefits of exercise—regular and at right intensity levels—for the immune system include increased immune-vigilance and improved immune competence, which help in the control of pathogens, a fact that becomes more important considering the immune-senescence and susceptibility of the elderly population to severe infections. Other favorable effects in relation to host factors, such as prevention or reduction of overweight, increased physical and cardiopulmonary conditioning, attenuation of the systemic pro-inflammatory and pro-thrombotic states, decrease in oxidative stress, improvements in glycemic, insulinic and lipidic metabolisms, besides the enhancement of the vaccination response, also show how adequately physical activity can help the organism's immune response against diseases.

CHAPTER 6

## Sleep

"A good laugh and a long sleep are the best cures in the doctor's book." _ Irish Proverb

Sleep and the circadian system exert a strong regulatory influence on immune functions. Investigations of the normal sleep–wake cycle showed that immune parameters like numbers of undifferentiated naïve T cells and the production of pro-inflammatory cytokines show peaks during early nocturnal sleep whereas circulating numbers of immune cells with immediate effecter functions, like Cytotoxic natural killer cells, as well as anti-inflammatory cytokine activity peak during daytime wakefulness. Although it is difficult to entirely dissect the influence of sleep from that of the circadian rhythm, comparisons of the effects of nocturnal sleep with those of 24-h periods of wakefulness suggest that sleep helps in the extravasations of T cells and their possible redistribution to lymph nodes.

**The sleep–wake cycle and immune function**

Life is organized into rhythms. A multi-oscillatory system with cellular clocks, in many if not all cells of the organism, synchronized by a hypothalamic pacemaker - the supra-chiasmatic nuclei, regulates the circadian (~24 h) rhythm of body functions and behavior. The sleep–wake cycle can be regarded as the most prominent manifestation of the circadian rhythm. Sleep and the circadian system are tightly intertwined. In most cases, both act in concert to adapt the organism to the ever-changing demands of the solar day and to separate otherwise incompatible body functions in time. Thus, very robust changes are evident during the regular sleep–wake cycle not only with regard to physical and mental activity, cardiovascular function and temperature regulation, but also for immune parameters like leukocyte numbers, function, proliferation and cytokine production. Of note, most of these changes occur in synchrony with the sleep–wake cycle regardless of whether the active phase occurs during daytime, like in humans, or during nighttime like in rodents (with one exception, i.e., the release of melatonin). Accordingly, such diurnal changes occurring in immune parameters during the sleep–wake cycle can be categorized into two classes according to their peak times, i.e., rhythms exhibiting their maximum during the rest period and rhythms with a peak during the active period. Before we go into the specific contribution of sleep to immunity, here we discuss the changes in immune cell counts and function as they are normally associated with the regular sleep–wake cycle.

**The early resting period represents a pro-inflammatory state**

The nocturnal sleep period in humans is characterized by a profound down-regulation of the two stress systems, the hypothalamus–pituitary–adrenal (HPA) axis and the sympathetic nervous system (SNS), with a concomitant drop in blood levels of cortisol, epinephrine and nor-epinephrine. In contrast, mediators serving cell growth, differentiation, and restoration like the pituitary growth hormone (GH) and prolactin and (in day-active humans) the pineal hormone melatonin show a steep increase in their blood levels during sleep. In parallel, increases of leptin that is released by adipocytes are assumed to prevent sleep-disturbing feelings of hunger during this time. Despite their vastly different cellular sources, GH, prolactin, melatonin, and leptin exert remarkably synergistic actions on the immune system. They are pro-inflammatory signals that support immune cell activation, proliferation, differentiation, and the production of pro-inflammatory cytokines like interleukin IL-1, IL-12, tumor necrosis factor (TNF)-α and of Th1 cytokines like interferon (IFN)-γ. In contrast, cortisol and catecholamine generally suppress these immune functions in an anti-inflammatory manner, although some specific aspects of immunity may be supported by these signals. Of course, when experimentally administered, the effects of these hormones essentially depend on dosage and timing, and here only acute actions of these hormones within physiological ranges are of relevance. On this background, numerous experiments have shown a consistent and intriguing pattern of endocrine and immune rhythms reflecting an 'inflammatory peak' during nocturnal sleep whereas wakefulness is associated with prevalent anti-inflammatory activity.

Peaks of pro-inflammatory and/or Th1 cytokines during the rest period have been seen, often during the early slow wave sleep (SWS)-dominated portion of sleep, in humans as well as in animals on the mRNA and protein level in different tissues including the brain, adipose tissue and lymph nodes, but also in serum/plasma and in unstimulated as well as stimulated peritoneal and splenic macrophages and peripheral blood cells (Bollinger et al.). Whereas the boost in stimulated cytokine production during the rest period can be explained by the above-mentioned shift towards increased release of hormones with pro-inflammatory actions, the question arises why spontaneous cytokine release shows a parallel rhythm. What is it that triggers pro-inflammatory cytokine production throughout the body with the beginning of the rest period? A tentative explanation is that very different factors accumulate during the active wake period which can be collectively termed endogenous 'danger signals' like reactive oxygen species, nucleotides (e.g. adenosine triphosphate) and heat shock proteins (HSP) and are released as a result of very different forms of cellular stress like physical activity, metabolism, synaptic transmission and cell injury. The action of these endogenous danger signals resembles that of exogenous danger signals, i.e. classical immunological stimulants of microbial origin like lipo-polysaccharide (LPS), muramyl peptides and other toll-like receptor ligands, in that they stimulate the production of pro-inflammatory cytokines by APC. Pro-inflammatory cytokines in turn exert a positive feedback acting themselves as danger signals and, thus, eventually support the initiation of adaptive immune system.

In addition to the effects of hormones and danger signals, immune rhythms are regulated by intrinsic cellular clocks that have been demonstrated in peritoneal and splenic macrophages as well as peripheral Th cells and are capable of maintaining periodic changes in pro-inflammatory cytokine production for several days in vitro. Clock genes control up to 8% of the transcriptome in immune cells, amongst others, components involved in antigen presentation, phagocytosis and LPS, HSP and NFκB signaling. Accordingly, various other indices of immune function, like phagocytosis, activity of natural regulatory T cells as well as spontaneous and stimulated cell proliferation in peripheral blood, lymph nodes and spleen, have been revealed to display diurnal rhythms, also peaking during the rest period. Interestingly, in the latter study, blood levels of GH and prolactin correlated positively with unstimulated IFN-γ production and with the stimulated mitogenic response in rat lymph nodes suggesting an active contribution of these pro-inflammatory hormones to the rhythm in immune function. On the other hand, low sympathetic activity (as assessed by tyrosine hydroxylase activity) seemed to contribute to the high spontaneous T cell proliferation in lymph nodes.

Taken together, neuroendocrine rhythms with the prevalent release of pro-inflammatory hormones and a suppression of anti-inflammatory hormones particularly during the early SWS-rich portion of the rest period in combination with an accumulation of endogenous and exogenous danger signals across the active wake period and the intrinsic clock gene activity synergistically impact immune and non-immune cells to boost immune activation during the rest period. This pro-inflammatory function of sleep can be beneficial. Thus, sleep after vaccination can enhance the subsequent adaptive immune response like an adjuvant. On the other hand, the pro-inflammatory surge during sleep can also be detrimental as evidenced by peak mortality rates in mice when LPS is injected during the sleep period (83%) in comparison with injection during the active period (10%), a pattern that is similarly observed for mortality rates in septic patients.

Sleep and the circadian system are strong regulators of immunological processes. The basis of this influence is a bidirectional communication between the central nervous and immune system which is mediated by shared signals (neurotransmitters, hormones and cytokines) and direct innervations of the immune system by the autonomic nervous system. Many immune functions display prominent rhythms in synchrony with the regular 24-h sleep–wake cycle, reflecting the synergistic actions of sleep and the circadian system on these parameters. Differentiated immune cells with immediate effector functions, like Cytotoxic NK cells and terminally differentiated CTL, peak during the wake period thus allowing an efficient and fast combat of intruding antigens and reparation of tissue damage, which are more likely to occur during the active phase of the organism. In contrast, undifferentiated or less differentiated cells like naïve and central memory T cells peak during the night, when the more slowly evolving adaptive immune response is initiated. Nocturnal sleep, and especially SWS prevalent during the early night, promotes the release of GH and prolactin, while anti-inflammatory actions of cortisol and catecholamine are at the lowest levels. The endocrine milieu during early sleep critically supports (1) the interaction between APC and T cells, as evidenced by an enhanced production of IL-12, (2) a shift of the Th1/Th2 cytokine balance towards Th1 cytokines and (3) an increase in Th cell proliferation and (4) probably also facilitates the migration of naïve T cells to lymph nodes. Thereby, the endocrine milieu during early sleep likely promotes the initiation of Th1 immune responses that eventually supports the formation of long-lasting immunological memories. Prolonged sleep curtailment and the accompanying stress response invoke a persistent unspecific production of pro-inflammatory cytokines, best described as chronic low-grade inflammation, and also produce immunodeficiency, which both have detrimental effects on health.

# CHAPTER 7

# Stress

"Every negative belief weakens the partnership between mind and body." – Deepak Chopra

Since the dawn of time, organisms have been subject to evolutionary pressure from the environment. The ability to respond to environmental threats or stressors such as predation or natural disaster enhanced survival and therefore reproductive capacity, and physiological responses that supported such responses could be selected for. In mammals, these responses include changes that increase the delivery of oxygen and glucose to the heart and the large skeletal muscles. The result is physiological support for adaptive behaviors such as "fight or flight." Immune responses to stressful situations may be part of these adaptive responses because, in addition to the risk inherent in the situation (e.g., a predator), fighting and fleeing carries the risk of injury and subsequent entry of infectious agents into the bloodstream or skin. Any wound in the skin is likely to contain pathogens that could multiply and cause infection. Stress-induced changes in the immune system that could accelerate wound repair and help prevent infections from taking hold would therefore be adaptive and selected along with other physiological changes that increased evolutionary fitness.

Stress is difficult to define. What may appear to be a stressful situation for one person is not for another. When people are exposed to situations they regard as stressful, it is difficult for them to measure how much stress they feel, and difficult for the scientist to know if a person's subjective impression of the amount of stress is accurate. The scientists can only measure things that may reflect stress, such as the number of times the heart beats each minute, but such measures also may reflect other factors.

Modern humans rarely encounter many of the stimuli that commonly evoked fight-or-flight responses for their ancestors, such as predation or inclement weather without protection. However, human physiological response continues to reflect the demands of earlier environments. Threats that do not require a physical response (e.g., academic exams) may therefore have physical consequences, including changes in the immune system.

**How could stress "get inside the body" to affect the immune response?**

First, sympathetic fibers descend from the brain into both primary (bone marrow and thymus) and secondary (spleen and lymph nodes) lymphoid tissues. These fibers can release a wide variety of substances that influence immune responses by binding to receptors on white blood cells. Though all lymphocytes have adrenergic receptors, differential density and sensitivity of adrenergic receptors on lymphocytes may affect responsiveness to stress among cell subsets. For example, natural killer cells have both high-density and high-affinity $\beta2$-adrenergic receptors, B cells have high density but lower affinity, and T cells have the lowest density.

Second, the hypothalamic–pituitary–adrenal axis, the sympathetic–adrenal–medullary axis, and the hypothalamic–pituitary–ovarian axis secrete the adrenal hormones epinephrine, nor epinephrine, and cortisol; the pituitary hormones prolactin and growth hormone; and the brain peptides melatonin, $\beta$-endorphin, and enkephalin. These substances bind to specific receptors on white blood cells and have diverse regulatory effects on their distribution and function.

Third, people's efforts to manage the demands of stressful experience sometimes leads them to engage in behaviors—such as alcohol use or changes in sleeping patterns—that also could modify immune system processes. Thus, behavior represents a potentially important pathway linking stress with the immune system.

## Pathway between stress and immune system

If the stress response in the immune system evolved, a healthy organism should not be adversely affected by activation of this response because such an effect would likely have been selected against. Although there is direct evidence that stress-related immune-suppression can increase Vulnerability to disease in animals, there is little or no evidence linking stress-related immune change in healthy humans to disease vulnerability. Even large stress-induced immune changes can have small clinical consequences because of the redundancy of the immune system's components or because they do not persist for a sufficient duration to enhance disease susceptibility. In short, the immune system is remarkably flexible and capable of substantial change without compromising an otherwise healthy host.

However, the flexibility of the immune system can be compromised by age and disease. As humans age, the immune system becomes senescent. Therefore, older adults are less able to respond to vaccines and mount cellular immune responses, which in turn may contribute to early mortality. The decreased ability of the immune system to respond to stimulation is one indicator of its loss of flexibility.

Loss of self-regulation is also characteristic of disease states. In auto-immune disease, for example, the immune system treats self-tissue as an invader, attacking it and causing pathology such as multiple sclerosis, rheumatoid arthritis, Crohn's disease, and lupus. Immune reactions can also be exaggerated and pathological, as in asthma, and suggest loss of self-regulation. Finally, infection with HIV progressively incapacitates T-helper cells, leading to loss of the regulation usually provided by these cells. Although each of these diseases has distinct clinical consequences, the change in the immune system from flexible and balanced to inflexible and unbalanced suggests increased vulnerability to stress-related immune deregulation; furthermore, deregulation in the presence of disease may have clinical consequences.

A decreased lymphocyte proliferation response is associated with increased levels of mortality and an increased number of hospitalizations among the elderly, but there is no clear link with specific diseases that are mediated by the immune system. Nevertheless, it is clear that stress has an adverse effect on health, probably mediated- at least in part -by the body's immune system. It is hoped that future research will show how, by reducing stress, we can improve health.

Modern medicine has come to appreciate the closely linked relationship of mind and body. A wide variety of maladies, including stomach upset, hives, and even heart disease, are linked to the effects of emotional stress. Despite the challenges, scientists are actively studying the relationship between stress and immune function.

In conclusion, majority of the research on stress and immunity revealed a negative impact of stress on immune responses. Research shows that both objective as well as perceived stress may negatively influence immune functions. The nature of stressor (acute or chronic) may have significant impact on the immune functioning. Brief acute stressors appear to enhance some parameters of immunity while chronic stress consistently showed detrimental effect on almost all parameters of immune functions.

# CHAPTER 8

# Vitamin A

"Keeping your body healthy is an expression of gratitude to the whole cosmos- the trees, the clouds, everything." –Thich Nhat Hanh

Vitamin A is a micronutrient that is very crucial in maintaining vision, promoting growth and development. It protects epithelium and mucus integrity in the body. Vitamin A is known as the vitamin of anti-inflammation because of its critical role in enhancing the immune function in the body. It is involved in the development and regulatory roles in the immune system especially in cellular immune response and humoral immune processes. It has demonstrated a therapeutic effect in the treatment of various infectious diseases.

It is a fat-soluble vitamin and insoluble in water. Vitamin A exists in the form of retinol, retinal, and retinoic acid, among which retinoic is the most prominent. The epithelium lines are the outer surface and most inner surfaces of organisms, and it functions as the front line of defense against pathogens invasion. Vitamin A plays a crucial role in the morphological formation of the epithelium, epithelial keratinization, stratification, differentiation, and functional maturation of epithelial cells. Vitamin A is the integral part of the mucus layer of both the respiratory tract and the Gastro-intestinal tract. Since vitamin A promotes mucin secretion, it improves the antigen non-specific immunity function of these tissues. It is shown that this vitamin improves the mechanistic defense of the oral mucosa, increases the integrity of intestinal mucus, and maintains the morphology and amount of urothelium cells.

Under conditions of vitamin A deficiency, epithelial cells shrink, and squamous keratinization may occur in skin, digestive tract, respiratory tract, genito-urinary system, cornea, and surrounding soft tissues, leading to symptoms of dry skin, diarrhea, coughing, dry eye, and urinary lithiasis. Simultaneously, the resistance of keratinized epithelial tissues to foreign pathogens decreases, and it is no longer able to exert its mechanical barrier function, thus reducing innate immune function and promoting respiratory tract infections, diarrhea, and other diseases of childhood.

Immune organs or tissues are places where most immune-competent cells proliferate, differentiate, mature, aggregate, and respond to immunity. It has been shown that crucial immune organs need constant dietary intake to maintain Vitamin A concentrations, and its role in promoting the proliferation and regulation of apoptosis of thymocytes. In the thymus, endogenous retinoid synthesis and retinoids like gluco-corticoids might, indeed, be involved in the regulation of thymic proliferation and selection processes, by being present in the thymus in functionally effective amounts. Vitamin A is also involved in the regulation of homeostasis of bone marrow.

Vitamin A is a very promising therapy for the treatment of IgE-mediated hypersensitivity disease. Regulatory B cells (B regs) are a class of B cells subsets with immune-modulatory functions of immune homeostasis and play an essential regulatory role in various immune-pathological processes. Retinoic Acid can induce the differentiation of naïve B cells into B regs, and stimulate synthesis and the secretion of interleukins which has shown beneficial effects on experimental colitis, arthritis, and lupus models.

# CHAPTER 9

# Vitamin B

"To keep the body in good health is a duty...otherwise we shall not be able to keep the mind strong and clear." - Buddha

B-vitamins are also very important in supporting a healthy immune system. For example, vitamin B5 (Pantothenic acid) promotes the production and release of antibodies from B-cells, and deficiency of vitamin B5 results in reduced levels of circulating antibodies in T-cells and can result in reduced effectiveness of the soluble factors as well. Vitamin B6 deficiency consistently impairs T-cell functioning and results in a decrease in blood lymphocyte counts. Deficiencies in vitamin B1 (Thiamine) and B2 (Riboflavin) may impair normal antibodies response and low vitamin B12 appears to inhibit phagocytic cells and possibly T-cells function.

Almost all whole grains, vegetables and fruits can serve as excellent sources of at least some of these vitamins, but some vegetables are particularly beneficial since they are excellent sources of many of these immune-supporting vitamins.

**Romaine lettuce** is a rich source of vitamin B1, B2, C and folate. **Turnip greens** and **spinach** are excellent sources of folate, vitamin B6 and Vitamin C. **Cauliflower** happens to be an excellent source of vitamin C, folate vitaminB6 and pantothenic acid. **Crimini** mushrooms are also an excellent source of vitamin B2, niacin and pantothenic acid. **Red bell peppers** are an excellent source of vitaminB6. Excellent sources of vitamin B12 include **sardines, salmon, tuna, cod, lamb, and scallops shrimp**.

# CHAPTER 10

# Vitamin C

"You can't control what goes on outside, but you CAN control what goes on inside." - Unknown

Vitamin C is an essential micronutrient for humans with pleotropic functions related to its ability to donate electrons. It is a potent anti-oxidant and a co-factor for a family of bio-synthetic and gene regulatory enzymes. Vitamin C contributes to immune defense by supporting various cellular functions of both the innate and adaptive immune system. Vitamin C supports epithelial barrier function against pathogens and promotes the oxidant scavenging activity of the skin, thereby potentially protecting against the environmental oxidative stress. Vitamin C accumulates in phagocytic cells, such as neutrophils, and can enhance chemo-taxis, phagocytosis, generation of reactive oxygen species, and ultimately microbial killing. It is also needed for apoptosis and clearance of the spent neutrophils from sites of infection by macrophages, thereby decreasing necrosis and potential tissue damage. The role of vitamin C in lymphocytes is less clear, but it has been shown to enhance differentiation and proliferation of B cells and T-cells, likely due to its gene regulating effects. Vitamin C deficiency results in impaired immunity and higher susceptibility to infections. In turn, infections significantly impact on vitamin C levels due to enhanced inflammation and metabolic requirements. Furthermore, supplementation with vitamin C appears to be able to both prevent and treat respiratory and systemic infections. Prophylactic prevention of infection requires dietary vitamin C intakes that provide at least adequate, if not saturating plasma levels (e.g., 100-200 mg/day), which optimize cell and tissue levels. In contrast, treatments of established infections require significantly higher (GRAM) doses of the vitamin to compensate for the increased inflammatory response and metabolic demand.

There is one enzyme by the name of L- gulono-lactone-oxidase, which is required to convert the last stage of six stage metabolism of glucose to L- ascorbic acid, and in humans and other primates lack this enzyme during the evolutionary genetic mutations. That is the reason we humans and other primates can't make our own vitamin c, which is fundamentally essential for the body to function properly. Other animals like goat and cow make their own ascorbic acid in the dose of many grams equivalent to humans during infections and stress period. When this mutation occurred, the humans and other primates compensated their vitamin c requirement from taking vegetables and fruits in their diet. In the modern world we forgot to take that quantity of fruits and vegetables due to all artificial fast and processed/packaged foods in our daily routines and missed the very important nutrient in our body so essential for our survival.

The deficiency of this vitamin results in a very severe fatal disease of scurvy, which is characterized by weakening of collage nous structures, resulting in poor wound healing, and impaired immunity. They are susceptible to fatal infections like pneumonia. This can manifest more in the malnourished population.

Vitamin C has a number of activities that could contribute to its immune-modulating effects. It is highly effective anti-oxidant, due to its ability to readily donate electrons, thus protecting important bio-molecules (proteins, lipids, carbohydrates and nucleic acids) from damage by oxidants generated during normal cell metabolism and through exposure to toxins and pollutants like cigarette smoke. Vitamin C is also a co-factor for a family of bio-synthetic and gene regulatory monooxygenase and dioxygenase enzymes. The vitamin C has long been known as a co-factor for the lysyl and prolyl hydroxylases required for stabilization of the tertiary structure of collagen and is a co-factor of fatty acids into mitochondria for generation of metabolic energy. It is also a co-factor for the hydroxylase enzyme involved in the synthesis of catecholamine hormones, e.g., nor-epinephrine and amidated peptide hormones e.g., vasopressin, which are central to the cardiovascular response to severe infection. It has also shown to act as co-factor in many more bio synthetic pathways like DNA and histone methylation and asparagines and prolyl hydroxylases actions.

The vitamin has crucial function within the skin. It is seen from the symptoms of the vitamin c deficiency disease scurvy. This is characterized by bleeding gums, bruising, and impaired wound healing. These symptoms are thought to be a result of the role of vitamin c as a co factor for the prolyl and lysyl hydroxylase enzymes that stabilize the tertiary structure of collagen. The anti-oxidant effects of vitamin C are likely to be enhanced in combination with vitamin E, which acts as anti-oxidant inside the cell whereas vitamin C acts as anti-oxidant outside the cell.

Leucocytes (White blood cells), such as neutrophils and monocytes actively accumulate vitamin C against a concentration gradient, resulting in values that are 50-100 to 199-fold higher than plasma concentrations. These cells accumulate maximal vitamin C concentrations at dietary intakes of ~100 mg/day, although other body tissues likely require higher intakes for saturation. Neutrophils accumulate vitamin C via SVCT2 and typically contain intracellular levels of at least 1 mM. Following stimulation of their oxidative burst neutrophils can further increase their intracellular concentration of vitamin C through the non-specific uptake of the oxidized form, dehydroascorbate (DHA), via glucose transporters (GLUT). DHA is then rapidly reduced to ascorbate intracellularly, to give levels of about 10 mM. It is believed that the accumulation of such high vitamin C concentrations indicates important functions within these cells.

The role of vitamin C is summarized below:

- Epithelial barrier function, it enhances the collagen synthesis and stabilization.

- It protects against ROS-induced damage.

- It enhances keratinocyte-differentiation and lipid-synthesis.

- It enhances fibroblast proliferation, and migration.

- It shortens time to wound healing in patients.

- Phagocytes (neutrophils, macrophages) Function: Acts as an anti-oxidant/electron donor.

- Enhances motility/chemo taxis.

- It enhances phagocytosis, and ROS generation.

- It enhances microbial killing.

- Facilitates apoptosis and clearance

- Decreases necrosis/NETosis (neutrophil extracellular trap)

- B- and T- lymphocytes functions: Enhances differentiation and proliferation.

- It enhances anti-body levels.

- Inflammatory mediators' functions: Modulates cytokine production.

- It decreases histamine levels.

Studies indicate that deficiency of Vitamin C is still relatively common in population. There are many reasons like reduced intake combined with limited body stores. Increased need occurs due to pollution, toxins, smoking, frequent infections, and diseases with oxidative and inflammatory components, e.g., diabetes etc. Ensuring adequate intake of Vitamin C through the diet or via supplementation, especially in groups such as elderly or in individuals exposed to risk factors for vitamin C insufficiency, is required for proper immune function and resistance to infections.

# CHAPTER 11

## Vitamin D

"Good health is not something we can buy. However, it can be an extremely valuable savings account." –Anne Wilson Schaef


Vitamin D plays important role in addition to its classic effects on calcium and bone homeostasis. As the vitamin receptor is expressed on immune cells (B cells, T cells and antigen presenting cells) and these immunologic cells are all are capable of synthesizing the active vitamin D metabolites, vitamin D has the capability of acting in an autocrine manner in a local immunologic milieu. Vitamin D can modulate the innate and adaptive immune response. Deficiency of vitamin D is associated with increased auto-immunity as well as an increased susceptibility to infection. As immune cells in auto-immune diseases are responsive to the ameliorative effects of vitamin D, the beneficial effects of supplementing vitamin D deficient individuals with auto-immune disease may extend beyond the effects on bone and calcium homeostasis.

The immune system defends the body from foreign, invading organisms, promoting protective immunity while maintaining tolerance to self. The implications of vitamin D deficiency on the immune system have become clearer in recent years and in the context of vitamin D deficiency, there appears to be an increased susceptibility to infection and a diathesis, in a genetically susceptible host to auto-immunity.

The classical actions of vitamin D are to promote calcium homeostasis and to promote bone health. Vitamin D enhances absorption of calcium in the small intestine and stimulates osteoclasts differentiation and calcium re-absorption of bone. Vitamin D additionally promotes mineralization of the collagen matrix in bone. In humans, vitamin D is obtained from the diet or it is synthesized it in the skin. As vitamin D is produced in the skin after exposure to UV B light, its synthesis is influenced by latitude, season, use of sun block and skin pigmentation. Melanin absorbs UV B radiation inhibiting the synthesis of vitamin D from 7-dihydrocholesterol. This initial vitamin D compound is inactive and it is next hydroxylated in the liver to form 25 OH vitaminD3. It is also an inactive compound but is the most reliable measurement of an individual's vitamin D status. It is converted in the kidney to the active compound 1,25 di -hydroxy vitamin D or calcidiol by 1-alpha-hydroxylase, an enzyme which is stimulated by Para thyroid hormone. 1,25 D acts on the intestine where it stimulates calcium re-absorption, and upon bone, where it promotes osteoblasts differentiation and matrix calcification. The active hormone exerts its effects on these tissues by binding to the vitamin D receptors (VDR).

Vitamin D has been used (unknowingly) to treat infections such as tuberculosis before the advent of effective antibiotics. Tuberculosis patients were sent to sanatoriums where treatment included exposure to sunlight which was thought to directly kill the tuberculosis. Cod liver oil, a rich source of vitamin D has also been employed as a treatment for tuberculosis as well as for general increased protection from infections. Vitamin D levels fluctuate over the year. Although rates of seasonal infections varied and were lowest in the summer and highest in the winter, the association of lower serum vitamin D levels and infection held during each season.

There is increasing evidence linking vitamin deficiency and auto-immune diseases including multiple-sclerosis (MS), rheumatoid-arthritis (RA), diabetes-mellitus (DM), inflammatory bowel disease and systemic lupus erythematosus (SLE). Vitamin D has also been shown to facilitate progression of existing auto-immune disease.

Vitamin D has many effects on cells within the immune system. It inhibits B cells proliferation and blocks B cells differentiation and immunoglobulin secretion. Vitamin D additionally suppresses T cell proliferation and results in a shift from a Th1 to a Th2 phenotype. Furthermore, it affects T cell maturation with a skewing away from the inflammatory Th17 phenotype and facilitates the induction of T regulatory cells. These effects result in decreased production of inflammatory cytokines (IL-17, IL-21) with increased production of anti-inflammatory cytokines such as IL-10.Vitamin D also has effects on monocytes and dendritic cells (DCs) it inhibits monocyte production of inflammatory cytokines such as IL-1, IL-6, IL-8, IL-12, and TNF-alpha. It additionally inhibits DC differentiation and maturation with preservation of an immature phenotype as evidenced by a decreased expression of MHC class II molecules, co-stimulatory molecules and IL-12. Inhibition of DC differentiation and maturation is particularly important in the context of auto-immunity and the abrogation of self-tolerance.

# CHAPTER 12

# Vitamin E

"It is health that is the real wealth, and not pieces of gold and silver." – Mahatma Gandhi

Vitamin E is a potent lipid-soluble vitamin, which is found in higher concentrations in the immune cells compared to other blood cells. It is one of the best known nutrients which modulate the immune function in the body. Its deficiency can impair the immune function in humans as well as in the animals and can be corrected with the repletion of this vitamin. The deficiency of this vitamin is rare in the humans but higher doses than the recommended supplementation in the elderly can enhance the immune system and can prevent many infections. The mechanism by which this vitamin works in the immune system is very much studied in cell-based pre-clinical and clinical intervention studies. Vitamin E is the common name of tocopherols and tocotrienols.

Vitamin E modulates the T-cell function through directly impacting T-cell membrane integrity, signal transduction, and also indirectly by affecting inflammatory mediators generated from other immune cells. Modulation of immune function by vitamin E has clinical relevance as it affects individual susceptibility to infectious diseases such as respiratory infections, in addition to allergic diseases such as asthma. Studies on vitamin E are mainly focused on $\alpha$–tocopherol; however other forms of tocopherols and tocotrienols are also known to have potent immune-modulatory functions.

The vitamin E being a fat-soluble vitamin and is most effective nutrient in its protective effect against oxidation of poly-unsaturated fatty acids which are enriched in membranes of immune cells, making them prone to oxidative damage is resulting from their higher metabolic activity and normal defense against pathogens. Smokers and athletes are more vulnerable to free radical onslaught due to excess oxidative stress and need more anti-oxidants in the form of vitamin E in their diet or supplements.

In human and animal studies, the role of immune-modulatory role of vitamin E has been demonstrated and is associated with reducing the risk for infectious diseases such as respiratory infections, as well as some allergic diseases like asthma. Respiratory infections, such as Streptococcus pneumonia and influenza, are particularly problematic for older adults as they are more susceptible to these infections, have longer recovery periods from infections and as a result have higher rates of hospitalization, morbidity, and mortality. Due to the vulnerabilities faced by older adults, both in animals and human studies main focus is given on the potential for enhanced immune function by vitamin E supplementation in response to respiratory infections.

Vitamin E also plays an important role in carcinogenesis due to its antioxidant role against cancer and against heart disease because of its limiting the progression of atherosclerosis.

Vitamin E is present in variety of foods and is fat soluble. When you consume it, you store it, you don't use. Vitamin E deficiency is rare in those who have a well-balanced diet. Those who consume a low fat diet may be deficient without intentional vitamin intake. There are several conditions and life-style factors that may lead to deficiency without appropriate intervention. Premature babies and people with malabsorption disorders are at the highest risk of deficiencies. Those who are immune compromised or have an auto-immune disease, may develop a vitamin E deficiency. A good nutrition is a helpful strategy in determining who will be at risk and understanding their individual needs.

Groups at Risk of Vitamin E Deficiency

- Pre-mature infants

- Individuals over 55 years of age

- Patients with Fat Malabsorption disorders

- Moderate to heavy alcohol users

- Liver disease patients

- Cystic fibrosis patients

- Lactose intolerance patients

- Crohn's disease patients

By eating a healthy diet, most adults will have their daily intake of vitamin E. However, deficiency can lead to decreased immunity, which is ever present on our minds now at this phase of pandemic. In tandem with immune consequences, long term deficiency of vitamin E can lead to serious health issues.

Symptoms of Vitamin E Deficiency

- Nerve damage

- Muscle weakness

- Vision problems

- Hardened arteries

- Loss of feelings in arms and legs

- Loss of body movement control

- Cancer

For these symptoms you can consult your physician and take supplements of vitamin E to boost your immunity and you can change your diet of rich vitamin E in your routine. Vitamin E is one of the 13 essential critical vitamins taken together promote whole body system health. There are a lot more health benefits of taking vitamin E, as it is particularly important in the immune pathways. Most people with healthy balanced diet get adequate vitamin E in diet but some may need to take in supplement form. Tocopherols are predominantly found in corn, soybean and olive oil and the tocotrienols are particularly rich in palm oil, rice bran oil and barley oils. Tocotrienols possess powerful anti-oxidant, anti-cancer and cholesterol lowering properties. Recently alpha tocotrienols is found to be multi-fold more powerful than alpha tocopherol in protecting neuronal cells from glutamate as well as other toxicities.

Foods with vitamin E

- Sun flower seeds

- Hazel-nuts

- Pea-nuts/Pea-nut butter

- Almonds

- Spinach

- Broccoli

- Tomatoes

- Mangoes

- Wheat germ oil

- Bell peppers Asparagus

- Avocados

- Eggs and fish

- Cod liver oil

Normally, a balanced and routine diet we can fulfill our daily needs of this vitamin but problem is with those who have some underlying problems of absorption and some serious diseases. Vitamin E is our potent modulator of immunity and it can save us from many serious illnesses.

# CHAPTER 13

# Obesity

"The problem is we aren't eating food anymore, we are eating food-like products." - FMTV-

There is strong evidence indicating that excess fat negatively impacts immune function and host defense in obese individuals. Obesity is characterized by a state of low-grade chronic inflammation in addition to disturbed levels of circulating nutrients and metabolic hormones. The impact of these metabolic abnormalities on obesity-related co-morbidities has undergone intense scrutiny over the past decade. However, relatively little is known of how the immune system and host defense are influenced by the pro-inflammatory and excess energy milieu of the obese. Epidemiological data suggest obese human subjects are at greater risk for nosocomial infections, especially following surgery. Additionally, the significance of altered immunity in obese human subjects is emphasized by recent studies reporting obesity to be an independent risk factor for increased morbidity and mortality following infection with the 2009 pandemic influenza A (H1N1) virus.

## Evidence of impaired immunity in obese individuals

Recent studies have demonstrated altered immune cell function in obese human subjects compared with those of healthy weight. Nieman et al., reported considerable discrepancies in leukocyte numbers and subset counts and phagocytic and oxidative burst activity of monocytes between lean and obese individuals.

Additionally circulating mononuclear cells in the obese exhibit a pro-inflammatory state compared with healthy weight persons. Impaired lymphocyte proliferation to polyclonal stimulation has been reported as well. Type 2 diabetes, a common complication of obesity, is associated with impaired immune cell activity. Individual s with a genetic mutation preventing proper synthesis of the hormone leptin, become morbidly obese and display weakened immune defenses. Interestingly, obesity has been shown to enhance thymic aging and reduce T-cell repertoire diversity, thus possibly impacting immune surveillance. The reported findings of immune cell dysfunction suggest that obesity may result in impaired host defense. Indeed, studies have linked obesity with increased risk of infection. Several reports have found obesity to be a significant risk factor for post-operative and surgical site, nosocomial, periodontal and respiratory infections.

## Mechanism of altered cellular immune function in obese individuals

It is well known that obesity is associated with a state of chronic, low-grade inflammation both in white adipose tissue and systemically. Additionally, obesity is characterized by altered levels of circulating hormones and nutrients such as glucose and lipids. Circulating immune cells and those, resident in peripheral tissues are thus exposed to an energy-rich environment in the context of altered concentrations of metabolic hormones. Understanding how this pro-inflammatory, excess energy milieu impacts immune cell function is the key in understanding the immune-deficient state associated with obesity.

Obesity is associated with a low-grade chronic systemic inflammatory state characterized by elevation of acute-phase proteins such as C-reactive protein (CRP) produced by liver and IL-6, secreted by adipocytes and adipose tissue macrophages, as well as by an increase in TNF-alpha by adipose tissue. Recent reports have observed higher serum TNF-alpha among obese subjects. TNF-alpha has been shown to be mainly secreted by macrophages that infiltrate adipose tissue creating crown-like structures around necrotic adipocytes. The role of adaptive immunity in obesity has been partly described. B lymphocytes have also been found within CLS (crown-like structures) in human adipose tissue, although their role is not completely understood. In addition, adipose tissue from obese subjects has been found to contain an increased number of both CD4+ and CD8+ T lymphocytes, which also secrete pro-inflammatory cytokines such as TNF-alpha and IFN-gamma. Increased waist circumference has been associated with increased expression of the activation markers CD25 and CD69 in T lymphocytes from adipose tissue. Th 1 cells secrete IFN-gamma, a pro-inflammatory cytokine, and Th 2 cells secrete IL-4, an interleukin with an anti-inflammatory role. Peripheral blood mononuclear cells (PBMCs) have been shown to exhibit a pro-inflammatory secretory profile in obese subjects. Also higher levels of the activation factor CD25 in T lymphocytes and increased TH 1/ Th 2 ratios, correlated with insulin resistance assessed by the HOMA index, have been reported in obese subjects compared with lean or healthy overweight controls. BMI has been found to be positively correlated with CD4+ effector memory T regulatory (Tregs) lymphocytes in severely obese subjects undergoing bariatric surgery.

The role of innate immunity in the development of obesity-associated low-grade chronic inflammation has been well studied. Evidence indicates that despite the lack of an identified specific antigen, the adaptive immune system; also participate in the development of this inflammatory state and exhibits pro-inflammatory polarization.

Obesity is associated with a systemic low-grade inflammation state in which cells from the innate and adaptive immune system increase pro-inflammatory cytokines secretion. Among other potential mechanisms, the inflammatory milieu leads to insulin resistance and metabolic co-morbidities. Weight loss leads to significant changes in adaptive immune cells. Both CD4+ and CD8+ T cell counts are reduced. Th increases anti-inflammatory cytokine secretion, which leads to an increase in Breg cells. Anti-inflammatory cytokines, such as IL-10 and TGF-beta produced by B reg cells, inhibit the secretion of the pro-inflammatory cytokines IFN-$\gamma$ and IL-17 by T cells Furthermore, a decrease in the Th 1/Th 2 ratio is also induced after bariatric surgery-mediated weight loss, probably related to improved insulin sensitivity. After weight loss, immune cells develop stronger anti-oxidant capacity and reduce the level of lipid and DNA oxidation products. Oxidative stress is a known modulator of lymphocyte differentiation, metabolism, and proliferation, which improves after weight reduction. There are changes in metabolic substrate availability after weight loss, including glucose, succinate, and fatty acids, influence the adaptive immune response. Palmitate, specifically, has been shown to promote T CD4+ effector memory cell differentiation in obesity. Mechanisms involved in the weight loss induced changes in adaptive immunity include weight loss per se, caloric deprivation, substrate availability, and insulin sensitivity, fatty acid, and metabolite concentration changes. It is clear from all this that the obesity has a very major role in the immune system negatively and weight reduction positively.

# CHAPTER 14

# Iodine

"Life with God is not immunity from difficulties, but peace in difficulties." – C. S. Lewis

There is a great misconception that iodine's sole function in the body is to act as an essential component of thyroid hormones. The thyroid gland is not the only organ to concentrate and organify iodine. Evidence suggests there are many extra-thyroidal benefits of iodine including maintaining the integrity of the mammary glands, anti-oxidant functions, anti-tumor activities, detoxification, immune system strengthening, and protection against potentially pathogenic bacteria. Since iodine is essential to every cell of the human body and has several biological functions beyond maintaining normal thyroid function, a re-evaluation of "iodine sufficiency" is warranted. Thirty years ago, Americans consumed twice, as much iodine as they do today, but the average daily intake of 240μg is still above the reference daily intake (RDI) for iodine (150μg), which is nearly one hundred times less than populations consuming non-Western-style diets. Because the whole body, not just the thyroid gland, needs iodine, most Americans would benefit from consuming larger quantities of dietary inorganic iodine.

## Extra-thyroidal Benefits

Deficiency of dietary iodine causes a spectrum of disorders including goiter, hypothyroidism, mental retardation, cretinism, and varying degrees of other growth and developmental abnormalities. The world's leading cause of preventable brain damage is iodine deficiency. The World Health Organization (WHO) speculates that iodine deficiency disorders affect 740 million people worldwide and that nearly 35% about two billion, of the world's population are iodine deficient. In an effort to prevent deficiency-related disorders, the WHO and other world health policymakers subscribe to similar optimal reference daily intake of 100-199 µg iodine per day. While this amount has preventative activity, it may be far from the optimal amount. In fact, the optimal intake of iodine has never been determined. While the thyroid is known as the principal user of iodine in the body, recent biological research has discovered several organs that actively concentrate iodine including the stomach mucosa, mammary glands, salivary glands, thymus, choroid plexus, kidneys, joints, arteries, and bones. The lactating mammary gland and salivary glands concentrate iodine almost to the same degree as the thyroid gland does. Growing evidence now suggests iodine provides several extra-thyroidal benefits when consumed in larger quantities.

**Dietary Sources**

Even though dietary habits and iodine consumption of Americans have dramatically changed in the last century, the amount of iodine consumed by the average American is still considered sufficient by the Food and Nutrition Board of the Institute of Medicine. Extensive use of iodine in the dairy industry or as a dough conditioner in bread making is a thing of the past. For many Americans, iodized salt is the most significant contributor to their daily iodine consumption. However, over the last 25 years, salt consumption in America has decreased 65%. The consumption of eggs, which contain iodine-rich yolks, has also been reduced because of cholesterol concerns. Another study recently reported the significance of iodine lost in the sweat, suggesting previous studies have underestimated the implications of iodine loss during exercise. Unlike the amount of research done on electrolytes replacement, little has been done on iodine replacement in athletes.

Insufficient iodine intake and sustained loss have significant implications to overall health. The Japanese consume iodine in milligram quantities compared to the microgram amount consumed by Americans. Equally startling is that Japanese women, who have among the highest iodine intake in the world, have the lowest rate of breast cancer mortality compared to US women who have the highest. Japanese women who adopt a Western-style diet have higher rates of breast cancer than women consuming traditional Japanese diet. Compared to the US, Japan has a higher life expectancy and the world's lowest infant mortality rate. While no direct conclusions about the health benefits of iodine can be drawn from these data, they do suggest that increased iodine is not only safe, but may also provide additional benefits not obtained with current Western-style diets.

**Iodine Functions in Humans**

Iodine exists in nature in several inorganic forms including iodates (IO3), Iodide (I-) and organic mono-atomic iodine (C-I). Naturally occurring molecular iodine is rarely, if ever, encountered. Molecular iodine must be synthesized usually by reacting either sodium or potassium iodide. Tincture of iodine, the usual source of iodine for purposes of supplementation, may be made using either sodium or potassium iodide according to United States Pharmacopeia specifications. Both sodium and potassium iodide enhance the solubility of molecular iodine. There are also organic man-made forms of iodine that are extremely toxic and should not be mistaken for the forms listed above. Inorganic iodine consumed in large amounts is well tolerated. Several grams of iodine may produce acute toxicity, but this is a rare occurrence. The greatest amount of natural iodine is found in our oceans. Foods of marine origin concentrate iodide and have higher concentrations than terrestrial plants and animals.

In humans, the various ingested forms of iodine are reduced in the gut and are absorbed as iodide. Once in the bloodstream, iodide is transported throughout the body and, eventually removed by the thyroid gland and kidney. The thyroid gland takes up around 60μγ of iodide from circulation daily to use in the production of the thyroid hormones triodothyronine (T3) and thyroxine (T4). These hormones are synthesized, stored, and released from the thyroid when  needed. After binding to target tissues, the thyroid hormones regulate a number of physiologic processes, including growth, development, metabolism, and reproductive function.

In states of iodine deficiency, the thyroid enlarges, which increase its surface area and its iodine trapping efficiency. More severe cases of iodine deficiency can result in hypothyroidism and decreased fertility. A recent study of the mammary gland showed that iodine contributes to the maintenance of its normal integrity. As oppose to the thyroid gland, which selectively accumulates iodide, the mammary gland favors iodine, suggesting that different chemical forms of iodine exhibit different functions in various organs. In human breast carcinoma tissue, iodine levels are significantly lower than in surrounding tissue in the breast containing the tumor. Fibrocystic breast disease (FBD) is characterized by micro cysts, fibrosis, epithelial hyperplasia, and painful lumpy breast in reproductive aged women.

Studies show iodine, rather than iodide, is the preferred form of iodine to support breast health. In addition to forming thyroid hormones, iodine in thyroid and mammary tissue can be incorporate into lipid molecules, called iodo-lipids, which regulate cell metabolism and proliferation and possibly have an anti-proliferative role in breast tissue

**Anti-oxidant and Anti-tumor Effects of Iodine**

The anti-oxidant properties of inorganic iodine were first revealed in kelp, when it was shown to neutralize hydrogen peroxide and prevent hydroxyl radical formation. The researcher also noted that kelp absorbed increased amounts of iodine when placed under oxidative stress. In cells, iodide can act as an electron donor in the presence of hydrogen peroxide and peroxidase enzymes to prevent free radical formation. Iodine atoms, iodinate, amino acids, lipids, and other membrane or nuclear components making them less reactive to free oxygen radicals. In mammals dietary iodides have shown anti-oxidant activity in the eyes, an ability to defend brain cells from lipid per-oxidation, and an increased anti- oxidant status of human serum. Iodine has also been shown to induce apoptosis in cancer cells both in vivo and vitro. The administration of iodine-rich kelp was found to significantly delay the occurrence of chemically induced tumors in animals. Human breast cancer and genetically modified lung cancer cell lines have been shown to undergo apoptosis in the presence of inorganic iodine. Studies suggest that high iodine intake is associated with lower occurrence of breast cancer, while lower intake is associated with higher occurrence of breast cancer. The incidence of breast cancer is three times higher in people with goiters resulting from iodine deficiency. Epidemiological studies have reported increased prevalence of gastric cancer in iodine-deficient Italian populations. With increased dietary consumption of iodine rich foods, these Italian populations have shown decreased incidences of gastric cancer. Researchers speculate this effect is due to iodide-concentrating ability of the stomach, which uses iodide's anti-oxidant qualities to protect the cells from damage caused by lipid per-oxidation.

## Other Functions of Inorganic Iodine

Additional benefits of consuming iodine in milligram amounts are currently being studied. Among these benefits is detoxification. In one study to determine the optimal dose of iodine, women supplemented with 12.5 mg. elemental iodine daily, and showed increased urine levels of mercury, lead, and cadmium after just one day. Although the exact mechanism by which iodine increases immune function is not much known, it has long been used therapeutically in various pathologies involving the immune system. Studies have reported that adequate iodine intake is necessary, for maintaining normal cell mediated immunity, suppressing certain auto-immune diseases, and possibly preventing the development of gastric cancer induced by abnormal growth of Helicobacter pylori. The long term consumption of high-iodide eggs resulted in increase lipid metabolism and thyroid function in animals. Long term consumption suppressed age-induced lipid peroxide accumulation in the brain, reduced serum cholesterol, and elevated tissue lipoprotein lipase activity, which accompanied a moderate hypotriacyl-glycerolemic effect. Aging animals fed high-iodide eggs also exhibited higher thermogenic and serum T3 responses to col, suggesting they were better suited to maintain normal thyroid function than control animals. In a small study of 12 patients with type 1 diabetes mellitus given between 50-100 mg of iodine per day, a decrease in the total amount of medications used to control the diabetes was seen in all patients, and remarkably, six patients were able to stop taking diabetes medication altogether.

Defining the Optimal Dose

Whole body iodine sufficiency may require consumption in milligram doses. The current RDI for iodine is 150 microgram per day. Although this amount is sufficient in preventing mental retardation, hypothyroidism, goiter, and cretinism in the majority of the population, it does not account for whole-body iodine usage. The RDI was last examined by the Food and Nutrition Board in 2002 and has not changed since 1980. While the RDI gives 1.1 mg per day as an upper limit of iodine intake, it considers only the body's thyroidal needs and not its extra-thyroidal needs. An iodine-deficient person can tolerate between 12.5-50 mg per day without reported adverse side effects, allowing enough iodine in the body to sufficiently cover all the needed areas.

Japanese population living in the coastal regions consumes copious amounts of iodine, averaging 13.8 mg daily due to the large quantity of seaweed in their diets. These people are among the healthiest in the world. The RDI of 150 microgram per day does not provide the body with sufficient iodine to create normal cell mediated immunity or to protect from gastric cancer and fibrocystic breast disease. The mechanisms for these extra-thyroidal roles of iodine are not well defined, but it is clear that iodine is needed in parts of the body other than the thyroid. For a generally healthy person living in any area, whether he or she has low or high levels of iodine intake, an amount of 12.5 mg up to 50 mg of inorganic iodine/iodide per day may support full body health. These larger amounts could enhance immune function and in women, contribute to the integrity of normal mammary glands. Although iodine is well tolerated, not everyone should take higher doses. Those who should not take higher doses include children under 18 and people with thyroid disease as the risk of subclinical hypothyroidism and auto-immune thyroiditis is greater in this population. It is imperative that anyone thinking of beginning iodine milligram dose supplementation be checked for underlying thyroid disease to evaluate for subclinical hyperthyroidism.

Americans consume only half the amount of iodine they did 30 years ago and nearly 100 times less than the Japanese. The number of Americans who are iodine deficient has risen tenfold in a 29-year span. With food manufacturers reducing the amounts of iodine in milk and breads, and the number of Americans consuming fewer eggs and table salt, many Americans are not consuming sufficient amounts of iodine. The recommended daily intake is 150 micrograms. This amount is far too low for many Americans. Even though this recommended intake reduces the prevalence of hypothyroidism related to iodine deficiency, it does not take into account whole-body health. Daily iodine intake in the milligram dosage may provide immune system benefits and anti-oxidant protection. Increased inorganic iodine/iodide has been shown to be safe in healthy adults whether iodine-deficient or not. The benefits of increased iodine intake may include improvements in fibrocystic breast disease, a decrease in gastric and breast cancer risk, and a reduction in the amount of medication needed to control diabetes mellitus. The anti-oxidant and ant-proliferative effects of iodine on the body may benefit healthy individuals.

# CHAPTER 15

# Fasting

"An ounce of prevention is worth a pound of cure." – Benjamin Franklin

Studies have shown that fasting can regenerate entire immune system. The effect can be obtained within three days. With fasting, the body starts producing stem cells which are then used to fight the infection. This property is now being used to test on immune-compromised individuals including those who have cancer or those patients on chemotherapy.

Fasting can be especially beneficial in the elderly whose immune system loses its effectiveness with age. When the body is fasting, it prompts the stem cells to begin proliferating and rebuild the entire immune system. The body is able to remove the parts of immune system which might be damaged or old. Multiple cycles of fasting can have tremendous impact in regenerating the immune system. Fasting also stimulates the body use glucose and fat stores and breaks down white blood cells. This breakage triggers the regeneration of new immune system cells.

In a research study, participants were asked to regularly fast for between two and four days over a six-month period. Scientists found that prolonged fasting reduced the enzyme PKA (Protein Kinase A), which is linked to ageing and a hormone which increases cancer risk and tumor growth.  Per the scientists, when an individual starves, the body tries to save energy by recycling immune cells that are not needed, especially that may be damaged.

Early clinical studies have also shown that fasting for 72 hours also protected cancer patients against the toxic impact of chemotherapy.

# CHAPTER 16

## Sauna

"The cells in your body react to everything that your mind says. Negativity brings down your immune system." – Loretta Lanphier-

Sauna therapy is one of the best strategies to boost our immunity. It can serve an easy way to benefit our health; you can get this while doing your routine exercises.

- Increases Growth Hormone (HGH): Sauna therapy has shown to increase HGH up to 5 times baseline levels.HGH acts to preserve lean body tissue, burn fat, improve cellular health and immune response.

- Reduces Inflammation: Sauna therapy improves the body's immune response and reduces inflammation.

- Activates Heat Shock Proteins (HSPs): HSPs act to break down damaged proteins and stimulate re-growth. Sauna therapy activates HSPs by up to 16 times the baseline.

- Stimulate Autophagy: Autophagy is when the body breaks down bad cells and recycles the components for cell renewal. Sauna therapy activates HSPs which enhance autophagy and cell renewal.

- Facilitates Detoxification: Sweating is one of the main ways we eliminate toxic chemicals like heavy metals and bisphenols

- Improves Physical Endurance: It improves cardio-metabolic endurance.

- Increase Blood Plasma Volume and Blood Flow: Total blood plasma volume expansion helps to improve circulation.

- Improves Thermo-Regulation response: Body becomes better at adapting to hot and cold environment.

# CHAPTER 17

# Deep Breathing

"If you know the art of deep breathing, you have the strength, wisdom and courage of ten tigers." - Chinese adage-

Over 90% of modern people suffer from breathing problems. The common problems include chest breathing, mouth breathing, and hyper-ventilation (increased minute ventilation). All of these factors reduce oxygen levels in the body cells and promote chronic diseases. Among the main causes of over-breathing in the modern population are drastic changes in diet and a lack of physical exercise with 100% nose breathing.

During the 1960-70's, the consumption of carbohydrates (both, sugars and starches) was dramatically increased, the Food Pyramid was invented and became popular, and dietary fats became enemies. This way case of obesity increased and there developed the problems of abnormal breathing patterns.

Dr Artour Rakhimov, an alternative Health Educator and Author, says that this is the most challenging health therapies since the students are required to make changes in their automatic (or conscious) breathing patterns in the right direction. While breathing more than the medical norm, most people believe that they have good or "normal" breathing. Some of them even say that their breathing is barely noticeable. But normal breathing is so tiny that healthy people experience virtually no sensations in relation to their breathing at rest.

The breathing technique is officially approved by one Ministry of Health and BTS (British Thoracic Society) to treat asthma. In fact, in 2015 the BTS provided an A++ score to this breathing technique for the treatment of asthma.

This is far better than meditation, any yoga modality, or any other alternative health option. The team of over 150 medical doctors also had successful clinical pilot trials (approbations) of the same therapy on people with hypertension, radiation disease, hepatitis B, liver cirrhosis, and even HIV-AIDS.

Benefits of deep diaphragmatic breathing are shown in many research papers worldwide. The air we breathe converts into chemicals that we need to fuel our cells. The way we breathe matters and even impacts our body chemistry. But how do our breathing habits influence our immunity?

## Inflammation

A study from 2005 discussed the potential for sudarshan kriya and pranayam breathing processes, forms of rhythmic breathing, in immune system improvements and stress reduction.

What's interesting is that cancer patients were the subject of study and the results showed that: performing regular breathing exercises could help boost immune cells that can combat cancer progressions.

The study looked at what's called natural killer cells (NK) a type of cell critical to the body's immune system. And found that controlled rhythmic breathing increased NK cells over a 3 to 6-month period. It's not a quick fix, but it's a positive step in the right direction.

## Breathing and Autoimmune response

Controlled breathing has a positive effect on the body by:

- Lowering cortisol levels

- Lowering blood pressure

- Improving autonomic (the automatic system in our body that works behind the scene) response to physical and mental stress.

- Improving arterial blood flow

Taken together, these elements add up to a powerful disease-fighting box of tools. Mindful breathing can help fight the progression of auto-immune diseases by bringing our body back into the calm part of our nervous system, the parasympathetic system.

Cortisol is often called the body's stress hormone. It performs many functions; too many to go into here, but know that high cortisol levels are bad thing. High cortisol is associated with auto-immune diseases, poor sleep, hormone imbalance and so much more and a good enough reason, to keep this stress hormone in check.

## Slow deep breathing increases parasympathetic activity

One of the best ways to turn down the stress response in the body and activate the parasympathetic response is to use slow, relaxed, diaphragmatic breathing. The physiological responses to deep, controlled, mindful breathing are so profound that if we could bottle them and sell them as drugs they'd be worth a fortune. Fortunately for you, it's not that complicated... And it's free. Just breathe!

The immune function and auto-immune disease are complex topics. The state of our health is not black and white, nor can one-stop solutions affect it. A holistic approach to health will always win against quick fixes. Once we understand that improvements in these essential body systems can happen thanks to natural processes, we can take steps towards building a solid foundation for health. It's simpler than we think.

Learn to exhale, activate your diaphragm, breathe deeply, and work on fixing your posture. Simply thinking about better breathing will trigger positive immune responses. When we slow our breathing and reset our bad breathing habits we send signals to our body that all is well.

Breathing deeply and mindfully is one of the most effective things you can do right now for your well-being. You can consult the breath effect.

**How to choose proper breathing technique?**

Proper respiratory exercises should satisfy certain criteria in order to be useful for the health of the breathing retraining student. One of the things to consider is that the general approach of any breath technique should take our 24/7 automatic or unconscious breathing pattern into consideration, and not only suggests doing some breathing exercises.

In other words, what is the point of doing respiratory exercises, if you sleep with your mouth open and on your back every night? One can practice the best breathing exercises for several hours every day, but one can still die from the advance of cancer, heart disease, diabetes, asthma, bronchitis, or other chronic diseases due to the Sleep Heavy Breathing Effect, which is the main triggering factor leading to acute episodes (exacerbations) and deaths in the severely sick.

# CHAPTER 18

# Magnesium

"Remain calm, because peace equals power." – Joyce Meyer-

Magnesium is an important element and is not well recognized for its very important actions for the body. It is also important for the body's immune system. Many studies have been performed to prove the link between magnesium and the immune system, as well as its role in many biological functions, from controlling enzyme activation to regulating cell cycle progression. Magnesium is one of the most valuable micro-nutrients in the body, and there is a very strong correlation between magnesium and immune system.

Magnesium is required for both specific and nonspecific immune responses, otherwise known as acquired and innate immune response. Scientists have found connections between dietary magnesium and immune cell populations, as well as inflammation. It is a co-factor for immune cell adherence, C3 convertase, immunoglobulin synthesis, anti-body dependent cytolysis, macrophage responses and IgM lymphocyte binding. Does magnesium help your immune system? Absolutely, and likely more ways than you expect. Magnesium not only helps keep the immune system strong; it supports everyday bodily functions.

Consider magnesium for the proper function of the immune system and for supporting stronger immunity and boosting the body's defense systems. It is possible to use magnesium for immune support, and there have been plenty of studies that demonstrate the connection between the two. In studies, both cortisol and adrenaline production were associated with magnesium deficiency; these hormones lead to anxiety and additional pressure on the body, which impact the immune system's ability to function.

To help the body fight off illness, it's vital to get enough sleep. Magnesium plays a key role in sleep quality, as well. Studies reveal that magnesium promotes restful sleep because it activates the parasympathetic nervous system, allowing you to feel relaxed and calm. Another study discusses the possibility of decreased vitamin C absorption in the body when magnesium levels are low. And vitamin C is a critical component of optimal immune health.

There is also evidence that exercise can deplete magnesium stores in the body. When this occurs, energy metabolism is impaired, muscle function decreases and oxygen uptake is diminished, and electrolyte balance is affected. All of these conditions compromise the immune system.

By adding magnesium to your diet or supplement regimen, you can help boost your immune response and aid the proper function of your bodily systems.

**Best Dose to Support Immunity**

Most adults require between 350 to 400 mg of magnesium each day. It's advised to get as much of that magnesium as possible through your diet. By ensuring you get this much magnesium each day, you are taking positive steps toward boosting your immune system. To accomplish this, add more magnesium rich foods such as:

- Avocados

- Legumes

- Leafy greens

- Dark chocolate

- Seeds

- Nuts

- Whole grains

If you struggle with getting enough magnesium through your diet, you can add a supplement. It's recommended that you start with a lower dose to begin and slowly work your way up as you need it.

**How much magnesium is too much? And is there such a thing?**

Working from the Recommended Daily Allowance (RDA) of magnesium, we know that most people should consume. Others might benefit from a higher magnesium dosage, if your levels are extremely depleted; it's possible to up your dose. In fact, one study monitored participants that took 1400 mg of magnesium per day and didn't suffer adverse side effects.

If you are unsure what the appropriate magnesium supplement dosage is for your situation, it's best to speak to your health care provider.

# CHAPTER 19

## Cancer

"Healthy citizens are the greatest asset any country can have." – Winston Churchill-

The immune system in our body acts like our Defense Force to defend ourselves from external and internal invaders of disease and toxins. Some parts of the immune system look for unhealthy cells or something foreign to the body some send messages to other cells in the body about an attack and others work to attack and destroy micro-organisms that cause infections – like bacteria, viruses, fungi, parasites – or unhealthy cells. When the immune system is defending the body against infection and disease, it is called the immune response.

The immune system is made up of cells and organs that work together to protect the body and respond to infection and disease. These cells are in the form of Lymphocytes, which are white blood cells of the blood and the lymphatic system. They attack viruses, bacteria and other foreign invaders. There are other different types of blood cells but Lymphocytes have the most important role in the immune response. Lymphocytes are also called immune cells. T cells (also called T Lymphocytes) destroy damaged and infected cells in the body and tell B cells to make anti-bodies. B cells (also called B Lymphocytes) can turn into plasma cells that make anti-bodies that help fight infection and disease. B cells can also remember the types of infection and disease the body has fought against in the past. If the same germ gets into the body, B cells quickly make more anti-bodies to help fight it so you don't get sick. Natural Killer cells attack cancer cells or cells that are infected with a virus. Anti-bodies (also called immune-globulins) are proteins made by B cells that have turned into plasma cells. Anti-bodies travel around in the blood. They fight infection and defend the body against harmful foreign substances by recognizing and binding a substance (like germ) that is causing the body to have an immune response. The foreign substances or germs that anti-bodies bind to are called antigens. A specific anti-body is made by plasma cells to fight a specific antigen. An anti-body binds to an antigen like a lock and key. So only an anti-body made against a specific antigen can bind to it, much like a key can only open a specific lock. When this happens, white blood cells can find and destroy the substance that is causing an infection or disease.

**Antigen-Anti-body Reaction**

When anti-body binds to the antigen, this process is called this reaction.

The Bone Marrow is the soft, spongy area inside of most bones, where blood cells are made. Many of the blood cells in the bone marrow are not fully developed (are immature) and are called stem cells. Stem cells change and grow into different types of cells, including blood cells. Most blood cells grow and mature in the bone marrow. Most blood cells leave the bone marrow and move into the circulating blood and other areas of the body, like the lymph nodes and tonsils, once they are mature.

The Lymphatic system is the group of tissues and organs that make and store cells that fight infection and disease. The lymphatic system includes the tonsils, spleen, thymus, lymph nodes, lymph vessels and bone marrow.

The skin and mucous membranes are the body's first line of defense against infection and disease. The skin prevents most germs from getting into the body. But a cut or burn on the skin can allow germs to get in. Germs can also get in the body through any opening in the body, such as the mouth, nose, throat, anus or vagina. Mucous membranes that line parts of these openings help to protect the body. Cells of the mucous membranes are acidic, which also helps prevent infection from bacteria and other micro-organisms.

## The immune system and cancer

Cancers of the immune system include lymphomas and leukemia, which are also types of blood cancer. But all types of cancer affect the body's immune system. Cancer cells develop from our own cells, so our immune system doesn't always know that it should attack them. Sometimes the immune system knows that cancer cells shouldn't be there, but more often our immune system doesn't notice cancer cells. Cancer cells can even turn off the immune responses so that the immune cells don't attack them. Also people with cancer often have a weakened immune system. The immune system gets weakened when the cancer itself or cancer treatment, like chemotherapy or radiation therapy, affects the bone marrow. Blood cells are made in the bone marrow and when it is affected with cancer or its treatment, the numbers of blood cells that are made are lower than normal. When blood cell count is low, the body can't fight off an infection very well.

## Cancer treatments and the immune system

Certain drugs can help the immune system fight cancer. Treatment using these drugs is called immunotherapy. Immunotherapy works by boosting the body's immune response or helping the immune system to recognize and fight cancer. A stem cell transplant (also called a bone marrow transplant) replaces the body's immune cells. These are the blood cells made in the bone marrow that fight infection and disease. Stem cells transplant is mainly used in the treatment of cancer that affects blood cells, like leukemia, lymphoma and multiple myeloma. But stem cell transplants are also sometimes used in the treatment of other types of cancer including testicular cancer, retinoblastoma and neuroblastoma. The goal of a stem cell transplant is to get the body back to being able to make healthy blood cells, like lymphocytes, which play an important role in our immune system.

## How cancer starts, grows and spreads?

Our bodies are made up of trillions of cells grouped to form tissues and organs. Genes inside the nucleus of each cell tell it when to grow work, divide and die. Normally, our cells follow these instructions and we stay healthy. But when there is a change in our DNA or damage to it, a gene can mutate. Mutated genes don't work properly because the instructions in their DNA get mixed up. This can cause cells that should be resting to divide and grow out of control, which can lead to cancer.

**How does cancer start?**

When genes work properly, they tell the cells when it is the right time to grow and divide. When cells divide, they make exact copies of themselves. One cell divide into two identical cells, then two cells divide into four and so on. In adults, cells normally grow and divide to make more cells only when the body needs them, such as to replace aging or damaged cells. But cancer cells are different. Cancer cells have gene mutations that turn the cell from a normal cell into a cancer cell. These gene mutations may be inherited, develop over time as we get older and genes wear out, or develop if we are around something that damages our genes, like cigarettes smoke, alcohol or ultra-violet (UV) radiations from the Sun. A cancer cell doesn't act like a normal cell. It starts to grow and divide out of control instead of dying when it should. They also don't mature as much as normal cells so they stay immature. Although there are many different types of cancer, they all start because of cells that are growing abnormally and out of control. Cancer can start in any cell in the body.

**How does cancer grow?**

Gene mutation in cancer cells interfere with the normal instructions in a cell and can cause it to grow out of control or not die when it should. A cancer can continue to grow because cancer cells act differently than normal cells. Cancer cells are different from normal cells because they:

- Divide out of control

- Are immature and don't develop into mature cells with specific jobs

- Avoid the immune system

- Ignore signals that tell them to stop dividing or to die when they should

- Don't stick together very well and can spread to other parts of the body through blood or lymphatic system

- Grow into and damage tissues and organs

As cancer cells divide, a tumor will develop and grow. Cancer cells have the same needs as normal cells. They need a blood supply to bring oxygen and nutrients to grow and survive. When a tumor is very small, it can easily grow, and it gets oxygen and nutrients from nearby blood vessels. But as a tumor grows, it needs more blood to bring oxygen and other nutrients to the cancer cells. Cancer cells send signals for a tumor to make new vessels. This is called angiogenesis and it is one of the reasons that tumors grow and get bigger. It also allows cancer cells to get into the blood and spread more easily to other parts of the body. There is a lot of research that is looking at using drugs that stop blood vessel growth (called angiogenesis inhibitors), causing a tumor to stop growing and even shrink.

**How does cancer spread?**

As a tumor gets bigger, cancer cells can spread to surrounding tissues and structures by pushing on normal tissue beside the tumor. Cancer cells also make enzymes that break down normal cells and tissues as they grow. Cancer that grows into nearby tissue is called local invasion or invasive cancer. Cancer can also spread from where it first started to other parts of the body. This process is called metastasis. Cancer cells can metastasize when they break away from the tumor and travel to new location in the body through the blood or lymphatic system.

**Where cancer can spread and staging?**

Most cancers have a tendency to spread to certain areas of the body. This has helped doctors develop staging system that are used to classify cancers based on information about where the cancer is in the body and if it has spread from where it started. Many cancers follow a staging system from 1 to 4 that are usually given in Roman numerals I, II, III, IV. Knowing how a cancer spreads and where a cancer may spread helps doctors predict how the cancer will grow. This also helps them plan treatment and give appropriate supportive care. Cancer can spread anywhere in the body, but it's most likely to spread to lymph nodes, bones, the brain, the liver or the lungs.

**Is it Cure or remission?**

Many cancers can be cured with treatment. But cancers that is thought to be cured can still come back even years later. Therefore some doctors prefer to say that the cancer is in remission. Remission means there are fewer signs and symptoms of a disease (such as cancer) or that they have completely gone away.

Many believe that cancer is a systemic disease and it can't be cured with local treatment, and can only be cured with holistic approach by giving the body enough raw materials in the form of supplements and diet to fight this deadly disease by making the body perfect in every respect of its immunity and its defenses.

# CHAPTER 20

# Autoimmunity

"The strength of your immune system, the balance of your micro biome and health of your gut are all deeply inter-connected."

Auto-immunity is the defect in any arm of the immune system that triggers the misdirected immune function in the body. It may be defined as a phenomenon in which antibodies or T cells react with auto-antigens. Auto-immunity induces auto-immune diseases. The immune system has various mechanisms to suppress the immune response to the self, and the disturbance of these mechanisms results in auto-immune diseases. The defect may be in the innate and complement arm or in the adaptive arm which consists of cell directed T cells or humoral side B cells. The defect in immunity may be under function of immune system which may be genetic or acquired. The defect may be over functioning of the immune system where hyper-sensitivity reactions take place. This defect of the immune system may be called as misdirected immune response of the body in its immune system.

Auto-immunity is the failure of an organism in recognizing its own constituent parts as non-self, which allows an immune response against its own cells and tissues. Any disease that results from such an aberrant immune response is termed an auto-immune disease. Auto-immunity is often caused by a lack of germ development of a target body and as such the immune response acts against its own self cells and tissues.

The cause of auto-immunity may be genetic predisposition, environmental factors or leaky gut. The leaky gut is the main source of modern day increase in the prevalence of auto-immune diseases. The leaky gut is the name given to the defect in the lining of our gut endothelium which is only one cell thick and separates our external environment of what we eat and drink, from our blood and tissues. If any toxin or antigen particle crosses the defect in this one cell layer to enter in our body our innate body defenses react to it and produce an immunity reaction. This defect in our gut lining allows the bigger molecules of our partially digested foods daily but our repair mechanisms of the body heal it there and then daily. The problems occur when the load of these unwanted toxins and undigested particles overwhelmed and the problem start creeping in. Just take the example of wheat, which has gluten in it. This gluten is antigenic to the human body if not properly digested in the gastro-intestinal tract (GIT). All the proteins are digested in our GIT to their basic components called amino acids. These amino acids are absorbed through these lining cells perfectly and these cells do not allow the bigger molecules of these amino acids called peptides to be absorbed. In the case of partial digestion the proteins are digested partially and these are not digested to individual amino acids, which make these proteins like a string of beads. These strings of beads remain in the form of 3 or more amino acids strings, which normally are not allowed to cross through the lining but when there is defect in the lining (Leaky gut) these poly peptides cross over and cause problems.

Our body reacts to these poly-peptides in producing antibodies against them which are present in our body. These poly-peptides also mimic the structure of our own body tissue cells as our body cells are also made up of these amino acids in sequences. Where ever these antibodies of these peptides find the same configuration protein part of these amino acids they strike against that and produce inflammation and this triggers the auto-immune process. This process goes on and the inflammation goes on increasing unless we repair that defect which becomes the primary source of that trigger. The auto-immunity can affect any system or organ in the body because all the organs are made of proteins with particular sequence of amino acids and the antibodies against those peptides find the antigen sequence protein part in our organs and cells where they can attack easily.

Auto-immunity can be organ specific or systemic. The organ specific diseases are Type 1 diabetes mellitus, Good pasture's syndrome, Multiple sclerosis, Graves's disease, Hashimoto's thyroiditis, Auto-immune pernicious anemia, Auto-immune Addison's disease, Vitiligo, and Myasthenia gravis. The systemic auto-immune diseases are Rheumatoid arthritis, scleroderma, Systemic Lupus erythromatosis, primary Sjogren's syndrome, and polymyositis.

**There are three stages of Auto-immunity:**

- Silent auto-immunity

- Auto-immunity reactivity

- Full blown auto-immune disease

Some examples of autoimmunity include:

- 70% destruction of myelin sheath in Multiple Sclerosis.

- There is 90%destruction of Adrenal in Addison's disease.

- There is 80% destruction of villi in celiac disease.

Most common signs of inflammation to know your baseline, show sub diagnostic indications like, anxiety, and depression, energy level, brain fog. Some lab tests for inflammation include hs-CRP and Ferritin level etc.

The treatment of this malady is very difficult in the allopathic conventional system of medicine where they suppress the immune system and there may be temporary relief of the problem but permanent relief is no where to find and the problem lurks in the body throughout the whole life of the patients. But in the case of functional practitioners, they see and find the root cause of the problem and treat it accordingly with a specific protocols and the relief may be permanent.

As we have already discussed, there are three root causes of this auto-immunity:

## 1. Genetics:

Genetics is mostly not under our control and works in about 8% of the cases. The genetic system is influenced by chemical, physical and psycho-spiritual inputs to the body. There are a system called epigenetics, which controls the genetics and change the phenogenetic process governed by the genetics. Our genetics works through our genes. Our genes are working under the positive and negative switches. The positive switch opens the phenogenetic pathway and negative switch blocks the phenogenetic pathway. These switches are under the control of our, this epigenetic system. So we can change the functioning of these genes with epigenetic means of good nutrition and positive life-style variations. And this way we can control our gene 92% times through our, this epigenetic system. Our biochemistry is equal to our nutrition.

"Each of the 100 trillion cells in the human being is a living structure that cam survive indefinitely and in most instances can even reproduce itself, provided its surrounding fluids contain appropriate nutrients" - Guyton A.

## 2. Environmental Toxins:

These toxins, we can avoid through our food, water, air and our surroundings. Microorganisms, parasites, malignant cells, allergens and toxins are all around us and our immune system protects us like umbrella in the form of skin, mucosal lining, lysozymes, phagocytes, globulins, cell mediated immunity, complement and interferon. Essential nutrients from food are the fundamental building blocks of the body and these are vitamins, minerals, carbohydrates, fats, proteins, nucleic acids water and oxygen. Deficiency of these can inhibit the healing process. The average auto-immune patients have at least 4 deficiencies, including vitamin D, vitaminB12, zinc, omega3 and water. For most nutrients serum testing has limited value.

Water, oxygen and sunshine (which give vitamin D and melatonin) are often not considered nutrients for the body by conventional practitioners. We also are very cautious about the medications used to treat the auto-immune problems which can cause vitamin and mineral deficiencies and those may hinder the immune system.

Iron deficiency is also very common in these patients which can cause

- Iron deficiency low RBCs.

- Inability to carry oxygen

- Reduced energy production in the body

- Fatigue

- Chronic recurrent infections

- Inability to heal

This deficiency can be known with the battery of blood tests of the body.

## 3. Leaky Gut:

This is the main culprit in the pathogenesis of auto-immune disease where we can act whole-heartedly and get very positive results in our malady. Gut integrity and dysbiosis is the hallmark of all gut diseases and after those auto-immune diseases. Our 70-80% of the immune system resides in the gut. Our gut absorbs digests, assimilates, destroys and eliminates toxins, regulates water and electrolyte balance, harbors micro biome, and connects and communicates directly to the brain.

Gut immunity works through:

- GALT (Gastro associated lymphoid tissue). This is the defense mechanism in the intestine.

- Tight junctions: these are the junctions between the adjacent cells of the intestinal lining, which get disturbed or there are gaps and there starts the process of leaky gut.

- Mucosal IgA: this is the globulin protein of the innate immune system which functions against the toxins and foreign invaders at the site of entrance.

- Friendly bacteria: This is the army of our immune system and carries our 70% to 80% immune system, 99% our micro-genome and helps in producing many vitamins (60% vitamin K, and 40% vitamin 8 BIOTIN) and neuro-transmitters.

- Stomach acid: this hydrochloric acid is very important for the first line of defense and digestion of essential nutrients for our body.

Leaky gut is caused by Chemicals containing toxins like plastics, sugar and pesticides, GLIADIN (gluten), GMO foods, Candida overgrowth, medications (NSAIDS, Aspirin, Antibiotics, Antacids), infections, aggressive exercise, stress and food allergens, additives, & preservatives.

Healing can take up to three years and you are to take the following steps for cure:

- REMOVE THE BAD: All food allergies, Toxins, Infections, Inflammation, People/ relationship.

- REPLACE AND REPAIR: Good bacteria (Probiotics), Gut nutrients to repair enterocytes, food nutrients, environment nutrients, sleep and sunshine, better relationship.

- RESTORE AND MAINTAIN: Healing phase, work on building solid foundation of health, exercise, rest, sunshine, purpose and love.

The treatment protocol developed by Jeffrey Bland, the 5 R program (Remove, Replace, Re-inoculate, Repair and Rebalance) recognizes that most inflammation comes from the gut. The goals of the 5 R programs which has been the mainstay of functional Medicine for treating all chronic and inflammatory illnesses are similar to the goals of the paleo- auto-immune protocol, which is why these two methods work so well together.

Let us take a quick look at the 5 R program and how each of the "5 Rs" compare to stages in the Paleo autoimmune protocol.

- REMOVE: means removing toxins in the foods, irritants to the gut lining, food sensitivities, yeast, bacteria, and parasites. In the Paleo autoimmune protocol this is equivalent to the elimination phase of the diet. This would be a great time in your treatment to consider working with a Functional Medicine practitioner to take a stool and blood test at this time.

- REPLACE: means replacing stomach acid and digestive enzymes. Doing this with food is easy. It is also recommended to add a shot of apple cider vinegar to water at the start of high-protein meals and to include bitter greens (such as arugula and endive) to stimulate your parietal cells to release stomach acid. If this is not enough, hydrochloric acid tablets and digestive enzymes may be helpful.

- RE-INOCULATE: means restoring beneficial gut flora. Many Functional Medical practitioners suggest beneficial probiotic supplements to replenish normal gut flora. This is the equivalent of adding fermented foods as suggested in the Paleo autoimmune protocol.

- REPAIR: means supplying nutrients to heal the mucosal lining of the gut and support the gut's immune function. This echoes the recommendation by followers of the Paleo autoimmune protocol to utilize bone broths and organ meats. This soothes and heals the gut lining while also supplying adequate nutrition for efficient immune function. This specific recommendation may be adequate for many patients, others, however, may need to add glutamine, zinc, L-carnosine, glycine, and DGL to receive the full benefit.

- REBALANCE: Rebalance is about paying attention to lifestyle choices- sleep, exercise and stress can all affect the G I tract.

# CHAPTER 21

## Positive Attitude

"The cheerful mind perseveres, and the strong mind hews its way through a thousand difficulties." – Swami Vivekananda-

Studies have shown that a positive attitude can improve immune system and help individuals live longer. Research study on 50 adults, aged 65-90 years, across two years showed that the older people who focused on positive information were more likely to have stronger immune system. Positive attitude promotes healthy aging. Older people can protect their declining health by focusing on the positives.

In this study, participants were shown a series of positive and negative photos, which they later asked to recall, and their immune function was also measured through a series of blood tests. Participants who remembered more positive than negative images also showed better immune functioning up to two years later. Per the researchers, "Participants who recalled more positive than negative images had antibodies in their blood suggesting stronger immune systems than those of their counterparts, who did not show this positivity in memory." It appears that by selectively remembering the positive, the older individuals are able to improve the functioning of their immune system.

Research has already shown that happiness provides many health benefits. These new studies are showing the influence of positive outlook. Someone who focuses on positive information may be better equipped to handle stressful situations, takes a more positive long-term outlook on life, and is likely to maintain positive social interactions.

It has been shown that the individuals with a family history of heart disease who maintained a positive outlook were one-third less likely to have a heart attack or other cardiovascular event within five to twenty five years than those with a more negative outlook. This was shown by Johns Hopkins expert Lisa R. Yanek, M.P.H., and her colleagues, who demonstrated that even in people with family history who had the most risk factor for coronary artery disease, and positive people from the general population were 13 percent less likely than their negative counterparts to have a heart attack or other coronary event. Yanek and her team determined 'positive" versus "negative" outlook using survey tool that assesses a person's cheerfulness, energy level, anxiety levels and satisfaction with health and overall life. Although a positive personality is something we are born with and not something we can inherently change. Prof Yanek says, there are steps people can take to improve their outlook and reduce their risk of cardiovascular diseases.

The mechanism for connection between health and positivity is not entirely clear, but researchers suspect that people who are more positive may be better protected against the inflammatory damage of stress. Another possibility is that hope and positivity help people make better health and life decisions and focus more on long-term goals. Conversely, studies have shown that stress can weaken immune response.

Other studies have found that positive attitude improves outcomes and life satisfaction across a spectrum of conditions-including traumatic brain injury, stroke and brain tumors.

- Smile More: A University of Kansas study showed that any form of smiling, including fake smiling, reduced heart rate and blood pressure.

- Practice Reframing: Instead of stressing about a traffic jam, for instance, appreciate the fact that you can afford a car and get to spend a few extra minutes listening to music or the news, accepting that there is absolutely nothing you can do about the traffic.

- Build Resiliency: Resiliency is the ability to adapt to stressful and/or negative situations and losses. Experts recommend these keyways to build resiliency:

  o Maintain good relationships with family and friends.

  o Accept that change is part of the life.

  o Take action on problems rather than just hoping they disappear or waiting for them to resolve themselves.

# CHAPTER 22

# Gratitude

"We can cure physical diseases with medicine, but the only cure for loneliness, despair, and hopelessness are love" – Mother Teresa-

Gratitude is associated with many benefits for individuals, including better physical and psychological health, greater happiness and life satisfaction, less materialism, and many other facets of life. Scientists define gratitude as a two-step process: 1) "recognizing that one has obtained a positive outcome" and 2) "recognizing that there is an external source for this positive outcome", While most of these positive benefits come from other people- hence gratitude's reputation as an "other-oriented" emotion-people can also experience gratitude toward God, fate, nature, etc.

Some psychologists further categorize three types of gratitude: gratitude as an "affective trait" (one's overall tendency to have a grateful disposition), and an emotion (a more temporary feeling of gratitude that one may feel after receiving a gift or a favor from someone). Most of the studies on this subject focus on trait (or "dispositional" gratitude) and/or gratitude as an emotion.

A growing number of studies suggest that gratitude may make people physically healthier and adopt healthier lifestyles. In a 2010 review, Wood, Froh and Geraghty wrote, "Almost no studies have been conducted into gratitude and physical health, and this remains a key understudied area of research" But the studies that do exist, mainly published since that review, suggest there may be a connection. A study found that when participants felt appreciation, an emotion related to gratitude, their heart rate variability, an indicator of good heart health, improved. Other studies have found that more grateful people: report better physical health, are moderately more likely to report engaging in healthy activities, are more willing to seek help for health concerns, and sleep better and longer. A study of people with heart failure found that people with higher dispositional gratitude reported better sleep, less fatigue, and lower levels of cellular inflammation, and a study of patients who had had a heart attack or chest pain found that patients who had higher levels of optimism and gratitude two weeks after their cardiac event also reported greater improvements in emotional well-being six months later.

A few studies have explored whether gratitude may be linked to benefits for patients with various other chronic medical conditions. In one study, chronic pain patients with higher trait gratitude reported lower end anxiety and better sleep. A longitudinal study of patients with one or two chronic illnesses-arthritis or inflammatory bowel disease- found patients with high trait gratitude at the beginning of the study also had fewer symptoms of depression; that was still the case six months later.

Finally, a recent preliminary study suggests that gratitude might help prevent chronic illness. This study found an association between stronger feelings of gratitude and lower levels of hemoglobin HbA1c, a biomarker involved in blood sugar control. High levels of HbA1c have been associated with chronic kidney disease, a number of cancers, and diabetes.

Daily feelings of gratitude are also associated with elements of well-being. A daily diary study found positive relationships between daily feelings of gratitude and feelings of both hedonic (related to pleasure) and eudemonic (related to meaning and self realization) well-being. Additionally, feelings of gratitude during one day were positively associated with hedonic well-being (though not to eudemonic well-being) the next day.

Other studies suggest that gratitude may live up to its reputation as "the mother of all virtues" by encouraging the development of other virtues such as patience, humility, and wisdom. In recent years, studies have examined gratitude's potential benefits for children and adolescents. For example, studies have found that more grateful adolescents are more interested and satisfied with their school lives, are more kind and helpful, and are more socially integrated. A few studies have found that gratitude journaling in the class room can improve student's mood and that a curriculum designed to help students appreciate the benefits they have gained from others can successfully teach children to think more gratefully and to exhibit more grateful behavior (such as writing more thank you notes to their school's PTA)

**Immune Booster**

Grateful people—those who perceive gratitude as a permanent trait rather than a temporary state of mind—have an edge on the not-so-grateful when it comes to health. It is shown that the grateful people tend to take better care themselves and engage in more protective health behaviors like regular exercise, a healthy diet, regular physical examinations. Grateful people tend to be more optimistic, a characteristic that researchers say boosts the immune system. In one study, researchers comparing the immune systems of healthy, first year law students under stress found that, by midterm, students characterized as optimistic (based on survey responses) maintained higher numbers of blood cells that protect the immune system, compared with more pessimistic classmates. Optimism also has a positive health impact on people with compromised health. In separate studies, patients confronting AIDS, as well as those preparing to undergo surgery, had better attitudes of optimism.

**Cultivating Gratitude**

Income level is by no means the only measure of satisfaction with one's lot in life. It has been shown that people who have faced losses early in life have higher levels of optimism. But some of this optimism can be cultivated. Some techniques are:

- Maintain a gratitude journal

- Create a list of benefits in your life

- Talk to yourself in a creative, optimistic, and appreciate manner

- Reframe a situation by looking at it with a different, more positive attitude

# CHAPTER 23

# Gut Immunology

"All disease begins in the gut." – Hippocrates-

Gut is the perfect place for an immunologist to work as 90% of all WBC of the body are in the lining of the gut. Our mouth is one of the most important organs in the entire gastrointestinal immune system. We must eat our food very slowly, so that the body recognizes the immunogenic capacity of the food and makes it tolerant to foods immunogenic effects.

Cow's milk has about more than 5,000 proteins, and one of proteins is like the one found in the body. Over time, after prolonged exposure to the milk protein, our body also starts to react against our own insulin and cause diabetes mellitus.

In another study, the components of Rheumatoid Arthritis knee was given orally to the patient and patient recovered from his symptoms. In another study, sublingual therapy made of pollen was given to patient, reducing the autoimmune response.

**What landscape does the mouth have?**

The mouth is one area of the body with the most amounts of bacteria, virus, and fungi. Today's world is focused on hygiene and has developed dietary practices which affect the composition of the gut micro biota. This limits the exposure of society to the pathogens which impacts the maturation of the immune system and disease susceptibility.

Defects in gut mucosal tolerance can lead to Allergies and hyper-sensitivities auto-immune diseases like Inflammatory Bowel Disease, Rheumatoid Arthritis, Type 1 Diabetes Mellitus and Systemic Lupus Erythromatosis. This can also alter the intestinal and respiratory micro biome.

Mucosal immunology: Majority of exogenous antigens (microbes and soluble antigens) make contact with mucosal surfaces. Mucosa's anti-inflammatory predisposition is which maintains, Allostasis.

Allostasis: Homeostasis is actually a dynamic process; respond to a pathogen and/or antigen and the return to a normal level.

There are similarities and differences between the systemic and mucosal immunity. Where the similarities are like both have Macrophages, DCs, T cells, B cells, Neutrophils, and NKs. Both have cytokines, chemokines and antibodies. The differences are where systemic immunity has the pro-inflammatory predisposition and its antigens are in the lymph nodes, the mucosal immunity has anti-inflammatory predisposition- Tolerance and its sampling from its mucosal surfaces.

Gut Immune System:

- GALT: Gut associated lymphoid tissue

- NALT: Nasopharynx associated lymphoid tissue

- BALT: Bronchial associated lymphoid tissue

- MALT: Mucus associated lymphoid tissue

It is all about numbers, more lymphoid tissue cells in the intestine than anywhere else in the body. More antibodies in the intestine than anywhere else are including the blood.

Physical barrier: Gut epithelial barrier including the stem cells in the crypts which are continuously renewed. There is a selective barrier where membrane pumps ion channels and there are tight junctions, which adapt to permeability which is affected by cytokines. It takes only 21 days to replace the gut with a new one.

GALT Gut associated lymphoid tissue have 4 components: Peyer's patches, Mesenteric Lymph Nodes, Lamina Propria, Intra epithelial lymphocytes

Peyer's patches: It is a patch of lymphoid tissue, its germinal centers found along the entire small intestine. Approximately 250 Peyer's patches are present. There is no afferent lymphatic to these patches, sample antigen arises from the lumen of the intestine and these take decision to make, whether to react or not against that antigen, memory of the cells work here.

Mesenteric Lymph Nodes: These are the largest lymph nodes of the body. These are the cross road between the peripheral and mucosal recirculation. Unlike peripheral lymph nodes, they don't require TNF alpha or TNF receptors to form.

Lamina Propria: (Mono-nuclear cells): There are lots of macrophages in it and these are bactericidal and anti-inflammatory and produce IL-10 cytokine. These macrophages ingest microbes without producing local inflammatory response. And these activate Lamina Propria's CD4+T cells.

4.-Intra-epithelial Lymphocytes: 80% of the plasma cells secrete IgA antibodies. The cells are mainly CD4+, 10% of them are Tregs. They produce large quantities of cytokines. Intra epithelial lymphocytes are out 20/100 absorptive and are decreasing in quantity distally. They have heterogeneous characteristic of NKs (Natural Killer Cells), Mast Cells, CD8 cells, Express CD3 (TCR). They do not go through the thymus gland.

**Types of immune responses**

Some auto-reactive T cells are deleted in the thymus. Remaining T cells must be kept in check. T regulatory cells (Tregs) are one way that auto-reactive T cells are kept in check.

**What do T regs do?**

Decrease all other types of Th cells (Th1, Th2, Th17,) these suppress Mast cells, Eosinophils, and Basophils. These promote an anti-inflammatory environment in the gut and throughout the body.

## T regs and Tolerance v/s Auto-immunity

In cancer there are increased numbers of Tregs in the body, and too few in the auto-immune diseases like diabetes, MS, Asthma, thyroiditis, Inflammatory Bowel disease etc.IL-21 may convert Tregs to Th 17.

## Th 17 Response

This response is normal response to bacterial and fungal disease like Candida, Staph, and TB. There is excess of this response in some of the auto-immune diseases like MS, Psoriasis, RA, and Crohn's.

# CHAPTER 24

# Strategies to boost immunity

In nutshell these are:

- Be grateful and remain positive.

- Prioritize good sleep

- Avoid sugar and processed food.

- Practice intermittent fasting.

- Consume immune supportive foods.

- Fresh air, sunshine and grounding.

- Regular movement and exercise.

- Good hydration and drink herbal teas.

- Optimize vitamin D levels.

- Take pro-biotic and digestive enzymes.

- Use vitamin C and zinc

- Use an infra red sauna.

There are multiple small changes in life style that can help improve our immune system as well as the quality of life:

**Relax and be stress free.**

Some stress can be a good thing. It helps your body get ready for a challenge. But if it lasts too long, that's bad news. Studies show it can weaken your body's defense system. Avoid it when you can. Make it a point to unwind and do things you enjoy. When in stress do yoga, meditate or deep breathe. With this your stress hormones optimize and you feel relaxed.

## Get Your Groove On

It doesn't just make you feel good -- it's good for you, too. One study found a link between a healthy immune system and how often you get busy. Those who made love more often had higher levels of a cold-fighting substance in their bodies. The body relaxes after the act due to the release of feel good hormones and stress is vanished.

## Find a Canine Friend

There's a reason we call them "man's best friend." Dogs and other pets aren't just good buddies. They also give us a reason to exercise and boost our health in other ways. Pet owners have lower blood pressure and cholesterol levels and healthier hearts. Dogs can help your child's immune response and make him less likely to get allergies. This may be due to the natural immune response of the body due to varied antigenic encounters in the environment.

## Build Your Social Network

We all know friends are important, but strong social ties can also have a big effect on your health. People with healthy relationships are likely to outlive those with poor social ties. Want to broaden your circle? Volunteer, take a class, or join a group that interests you. And nurture the bonds you already have. In the centenarian club the social tribe interaction is one of the major longevity factors amongst them.

## Look at the Positive Side

When you think good thoughts, your body's defenses work better. Want to stay in your happy place? Savor the things you enjoy. Look for a silver lining -- even in tough times -- and try not to dwell on the bad stuff. Your positive attitude will bring all positivity in your life. Always be in the present moment, forget about the past and never think about the future. If you think positive, your future will be positive according to the law of attraction. Believe in yourself and always have a positive self talk which will bring positivity all around.

**Have a Hearty Laugh**

A giggle or two is good for you. Not only does it make you feel better, there's no downside. One study found that after people laughed out loud at funny videos, their immune systems worked better. Laughing is a good exercise and laughing relaxes your tense muscles.

**Think About Herbs and Supplements**

Some of these products can help your immune system, but we need more research to authenticate them. Because they can interact with other medicines, let your doctor know if you want to try them. He can help you decide which ones are safe for you. Herbs like Basil, Turmeric, Ginger, Garlic, Black-pepper, Rosemary, Thyme and Sage are known to boost the immunity of the body. Some of these and their actions on our immune system are given at the end of this book.

**Move Your Body**

Exercise is a simple way to rev up your defense system. It can also ease stress and make you less likely to get osteoporosis, heart disease, and certain types of cancer. You'll get the most bangs for your workout buck if you do about half an hour a day. It doesn't have to be hard-core. Any type of movement can help: ride a bike, walk, do yoga, swim, or even play golf. Half an hour can be divided into 10 minutes thrice a day.

**Get a Good Night's Sleep**

Without it, your immune system won't have the strength it needs to fight off illness. Most adults need about 7 to 9 hours of sleep a night. To get better shut-eye, you need to stick to a regular bedtime schedule, stay active during the day, skip caffeine and booze near bedtime, keep the bedroom cool, and give yourself time to unwind at the end of the day. You need both REM sleep and deep sleep during night to get benefits of reparative sleep of the body.

## Cut Back on the Booze

Alcohol plays a major role in how we socialize and celebrate. But too much can weaken your defenses and cause you to get sick more often. How much is too much? More than two drinks a day for men and more than one for women. Alcohol is a chemical and our body is to get rid of this chemical. Liver is the organ to do this honor and have to pay a heavy price for that. That is the reason Liver diseases are so common these days.

## Kick the Nicotine Habit

Do your immune system a favor and give up smoking. If it takes you a couple of tries before you quit for good, hang in there! Ask your doctor for advice on how to make this major life change. Stay away from second hand smoke, too. This chemical is also very much responsible for heart disease, COPD, Metabolic syndrome and peripheral vascular disease.

## Wash Your Hands

Send those germs down the drain before your body ever has to fight them off. Use soap and clean, running water. Wash for at least 20 seconds. If you don't have access to soap and water, a hand sanitizer can help (unless your skin is caked with dirt and grease). Just know that it won't remove all the germs and other bad stuff. Choose one with at least 60% alcohol.

## Eat more whole plant foods

Whole plant foods like fruits, vegetables, nuts, seeds, and legumes are rich in nutrients and antioxidants that may give you an upper hand against harmful pathogens. The antioxidants in these foods help decrease inflammation by combating unstable compounds called free radicals, which can cause inflammation when they build up in your body in high level.

Chronic inflammation is linked to numerous health conditions, including heart disease, Alzheimer's, and certain cancers. Meanwhile, the fiber in plant foods feeds your gut micro-biome, or the community of healthy bacteria in your gut. A robust gut-flora can improve your immunity and help keep harmful pathogens from entering your body via your digestive tract. Furthermore, fruits and vegetables are rich in nutrients like vitamin C, which may reduce the duration of the common cold

## Eat the Rainbow Colors

Colorful fruits and vegetables are full of antioxidants. These nutrients guard against free radicals, molecules that can harm your cells. To get a wide range, go for oranges, green-peppers, broccoli, kiwi, strawberries, carrots, watermelon, papaya, leafy greens, and cantaloupe. All these fruits and vegetables are full of phyto-nutrients and are beneficial immune boosters.

## Eat more healthy fats

Healthy fats, like those found in olive oil and salmon, may boost your body's immune response to pathogens by decreasing inflammation. Although low-level inflammation is a normal response to stress or injury, chronic inflammation can suppress your immune system. Olive oil, which is highly anti-inflammatory, is linked to a decreased risk of chronic diseases like heart disease and type2 diabetes. Plus, its anti-inflammatory properties may help your body fight off harmful disease-causing bacteria and viruses.Omega-3 fatty acids, such as those in salmon and chia seeds, fight inflammation.

## Eat more fermented foods or take a probiotic supplement

Fermented foods are rich in beneficial bacteria called probiotic, which populate your digestive tract. These foods include yogurt, sauerkraut, kimchi, kefir, and natto. Research suggests that a flourishing network of gut bacteria can help your immune cells differentiate between normal, healthy cells and harmful invader organisms.

## Limit added sugars

Emerging research suggests that added sugars and refined carbohydrates may contribute disproportionately to overweight and obesity. Obesity may likewise increase your risk of getting sick. According to an observational study in around 1,000 people, people with obesity who were administered the flu vaccine were twice as likely, to still get the flu than individuals without obesity who received the vaccine. Curbing your sugar intake can decrease inflammation and aid weight loss, thus reducing your risk of chronic health conditions like type-2 diabetes and heart disease. Given that obesity, type2 diabetes, and heart disease can all weaken your immune system, limiting added sugars is an important part of an immune-boosting diet. You should strive to limit your sugar intake to less than 5% of your daily calories. This equals about 2 tablespoons (25 grams) of sugar for someone on a 2,000-calorie diet.

## Stay hydrated

Hydration doesn't necessarily protect you from germs and viruses, but preventing dehydration is important to your overall health. Dehydration can cause headaches and hinder your physical performance, focus, mood, digestion, and heart and kidney function. These complications can increase your susceptibility to illness. To prevent dehydration, you should drink enough fluid daily to make your urine pale yellow. Water is recommended because it's free of calories, additives, and sugar. While tea and juice are also hydrating, it's best to limit your intake of fruit juice and sweetened tea because of their high sugar contents. As a general guideline, you should drink when you're thirsty and stop when you're no longer thirsty. You may need more fluids if you exercise intensely, work outside, or live in a hot climate; this statement is true only for young people. In old age, people do not feel thirsty even if they are dehydrated, because their sensations are blunted. It's important to note that older adults begin to lose the urge to drink, as their bodies do not signal thirst adequately. Older adults need to drink regularly even if they do not feel thirsty.

## (a) Turmeric (The golden spice)

A widely used food spice and medicinal plant. The use of turmeric dates back, nearly 4,500 years, in Indian culture. Derived from the root of Curcuma longa plant in the ginger family.120 clinical trials with 6,000 human participants conducted successfully for safety and efficacy of turmeric as of 2017. It is "Generally recognized as safe" by FDA. And contains >100 chemical compounds.

Active components in Turmeric include Turmerones, Curcuminoids, and Turmerones. Turmerones are volatile essential oils. They constitute 6% of turmeric. Curcuminoids are phenolic compounds. They constitute 3-4 % of turmeric. Types of Curcuminoids include Curcumin (CUR I), Desmethoxycurcumin (CUR II), and Bis-demethoxycurcumin (CUR III).

**Health Benefits of Turmeric**

Turmeric affects the health of following organs – Skin, brain, joint, liver, cardiovascular system, digestive system, wound healing, immunity, reproductive system, and metabolism.

Turmeric has following effects on the body:

- Anti-oxidant

- Anti- inflammatory

- Anti-carcinogenic

- Anti-mutagenic

- Anti-proliferative

- Cardio-protective

- Hepato-protective

- Neuro-protective

Most of the medicinal benefits of Turmeric are due to Curcumin. Curcumin affects ~100 molecular targets. Types of targets include: Enzymes, Growth factors, inflammatory cytokines, Kinases, Adhesion molecules, Cell surface receptors, Apoptotic regulators, and other molecules. Curcumin modulates immune cells and immune cell cytokines from innate as well as adaptive immune system through its Anti-oxidative and Anti-inflammatory properties. Curcumin mitigates allergy and asthma. Curcumin mitigates several autoimmune diseases and metabolic diseases through modulation of immune system.

Curcumin augments the cytotoxicity of natural killer cells against pathogens. Curcumin increase the activation of anti-inflammatory M2 macrophages' to mitigate inflammation. Curcumin lowers oxidative stress created by inflammatory M1 macrophages. Curcumin suppresses activation of pro-inflammatory cytokine IL-2. IL-2 is needed to proliferation of inflammatory T cells such as Th1 and Th17 cells. Curcumin stimulates proliferation of antibody-producing B cells through suppression of oxidative stress. Curcumin inhibits inflammatory enzymes such as COX-2 that produce inflammatory cytokines. Oxidative stress aggravates allergy.

Curcumin mitigates allergy reaction by reducing oxidative stress. Inflammatory cytokines such as IL-2, IL-5, GM-CSF, IL-4, are associated with bronchial asthma. Curcumin alleviates bronchial asthma by lowering the production of inflammatory cytokines.

Curcumin inhibits the inflammatory cytokines TNF-alpha and IL-1beta thereby lowering a beta plaque formation, a hallmark of Alzheimer's disease. Curcumin promotes anti-oxidant and anti-inflammatory environment thereby lowering atherosclerosis and hypertension. Curcumin lowers the density of inflammatory CD8+ T cells that are implicated in Psoriasis. Curcumin inhibits inflammatory cytokines IL-12, implicated in pathogenesis of Multiple Sclerosis

## Recommended Dose in studies

- Turmeric Maintenance Dose: 1 gm per day

- Turmeric for acute inflammation: 30 gm per day

- Curcumin dose for osteoarthritis: 500 mg Curcumin two to four times a day

- Curcumin dose for Cardiovascular Disease: 70 – 2000 mg per day

# (b) Cinnamon (Cinnamomum zeylanicum)

Cinnamon is widely used spice and is aromatic native to south East Asia. Medicinal use of cinnamon dates back to nearly 4,000 years in ancient of Indian and Chinese cultures. Bark (tree and root) and oil of cinnamon have medicinal values. Cinnamon has minerals, vitamins, Flavonoids, essential oils. It has calcium, manganese, potassium, phosphorus. Cinnamon also has Vitamin A, C, E; K. Flavonoids found in Cinnamon include Gossypin, Gnaphalin, Hesperidins, Hibifolin, Hypolaetin, Oroxindin, and Quercetin. These act as anti-oxidants and anti-inflammatory compounds. There are also 41 essential oils found in cinnamon. Major essential oil components with medicinal effects include Cinnamaldehyde, Cinnamic acid, Cinnamyl acetate, and Eugenol.

## Health Benefits of Cinnamon

Cinnamon has many health benefits.

- Lowers blood sugar levels

- Lowers cholesterol levels

- Lowers onset of chronic illnesses

- Reduces inflammation

- Helps in weight loss

- Boosts immune system

- Aids in digestion

- Boosts functioning of the brain

- Has antibacterial and antifungal effects

Cinnamon modulates immune response via anti-inflammatory mechanisms. Cinnamon is shown to be Anti-bacterial and

Antifungal. Micro-organisms do not develop resistance to cinnamon. Cinnamon active compounds inhibit enzymes such as COX-2 and iNOS that are involved inflammation signaling. Cinnamonols inhibit transcription factor NF-kB which is responsible for transcription of inflammatory genes that cause "cytokine Storm" such as TNF – alpha and IL – 8.

Cinnamon is effective against several fungi including Aspergillus flavus (Causes rot in grains), Aspergillus fumigates (causes allergic diseases), Trichophyton rubrum (causes athlete's foot), and Candida (causes genital and oral infections). Fungi do not develop resistance to cinnamon. It causes its affects against fungi through cell membrane disruption.

Cinnamon is effective against several bacteria including Escherichia coli (Causes diarrhea, UTI), Staphylococcus (causes Staph.), Listeria (causes Listeriosis), Salmonella (causes diarrhea), and Porphyromonas gingivalus (causes periodontal diseases). Bacteria do not develop resistance to Cinnamon. Cinnamon causes its antibacterial action by damaging bacterial cell membranes, leading to leakage of cellular content is and death of the bacteria. It also inhibits Z-ring formation, which stops cell division, and reduces the virulence of bacteria. It also inhibits ATP production, which leads to starvation of the bacteria.

**Recommended Dose in studies**

- Maintenance dose: 120 mg/day to 6gm/day

- For wound healing: 2% (w/w) cinnamon ointment

- For sugar control: 1 – 6 g/day

- For antimicrobial activity: 3 capsules per day are given, containing 18 mg Cinnamon oil and 9 mg pogostemon oil.

# (c) Black Cumin Seed (Nigella sativa)

This herb is native to middle and South East Asia. It is used in treating various animal and human ailments over centuries. The medicinal benefits are attributed to seeds and seed oil. Black Cumin seed has 62 compounds including Fatty acids, Minerals, Polyphenols, and Vitamins. It also has minerals including Calcium, Magnesium, Potassium, and Phosphorus. The vitamins in Black Cumin Seed Oil include Vitamin C, Vitamin E. The active compounds with medicinal benefits are found in black cumin seeds are Thymoquinone, Nigellone, p-Cymene, Carvacrol, alpha-Thujene, Thymol, and alpha- Pinene

**Health benefits of Black Cumin Seed**

Black Cumin Seed's health benefits include:

- Analgesic

- Anti-Bacterial

- Anti- Viral

- Anti-diabetic

- Anti- inflammatory

- Anti- cancer

- Immune modulator

Black Cumin Seed modulates immune response via ant-inflammatory mechanisms. Black Cumin Seed is shown to be Anti viral and Anti bacterial. Bacteria do not develop resistance to Black Cumin Seed. It also modulates inflammatory enzymes and cytokines. Inflammation leads to harmful and disproportionate immune response. Transcription factor NF-kB promotes the expression of inflammatory enzymes such as COX-2 and 5-LOX. Black Cumin Seed active compound Thymoquinone inhibits NF-kB thereby inhibiting expression of COX -2 and 5- LOX.

The Anti-viral activity of Black Cumin Seed is through increased production of IFN-gamma. Higher IFN-gamma increased the production of innate immune cells including Macrophages, and Cytotoxic T cells. Macrophages and Cytotoxic T cells directly kill the virus and mitigate the infection.

The Thymoquinone in Black Cumin Seed Oil has been shown to have a broad spectrum antibacterial activity. Thymoquinone exerts its anti-bacterial effect through inhibition of bio-film formation. A bio-film is a cluster of bacteria attached to biotic surface that allows them to survive in hostile environmental conditions. Thymoquinone inhibits the bio-film and kills the exposed bacteria effectively. It is effective against Staphylococcus (causes staph.), Listeria (causes listeriosis), and Porphyromonas gingivalis (causes periodontal diseases). Bacteria do not develop resistance to Thymoquinone.

**Recommended Dose in studies**

- Maintenance dose: 250 – 1000 mg/day of black cumin seed oil

- For inflammation in Rheumatoid Arthritis: 1000 mg/day black cumin seed oil

- For Anti- diabetic use: 1 – 3 gm seed/day

- For immune system boost: 2.4 gm – 4.8gm/day

Neem is mainly cultivated in the Indian subcontinent. It has been used as a medicine for more than 4,500 years. Its fruits, seeds oil, leaves, bark, and roots show an important role in diseases prevention. More than 140 compounds have been isolated so far from different parts of Neem tree. Most of the medicinal benefits are derived from two groups of compounds: Isoprenoids including Di- and tri terpenoids; and Non- Isoprenoids including Phenolic compounds

## Health benefits of Neem

Neem inhibits inflammatory enzymes such as COX 2 and 5- LOX thereby modulating the runaway host immune response. It activates adaptive immune cells to directly kill viruses. If used as toothpaste, the inhibition of dental plaque formation reduces bacteria. Neem kills bacteria and fungi via disruption of cell membrane.

Some medicinal uses of Neem as mentioned in the ancient medicinal text Ayurveda include:

- Leaf- Leprosy, eye problems, intestinal worms, anorexia, biliousness, and skin ulcers.

- Flower- Bile suppression, elimination of intestinal worms and phlegm.

- Twig:-Relieves cough, asthma, piles, spermatorrhoea, obstinate urinary disorder, diabetes.

- Bark- Analgesic and antipyretic

- Fruit-Relieves piles intestinal worms, Urinary disorder, eye problems, diabetes, wound healing and Leprosy.

- Gum - Effective against skin diseases, like ringworms, scabies, wound an ulcer.

- Seed pulp-Leprosy and intestinal worms.

- Oil- Leprosy and intestinal worms

- Root, bark, fruit and flower together- Blood morbidity, biliary afflictions, itching, skin ulcers, burning sensation and leprosy.

Neem is one of the most versatile naturally occurring medicinal herbs. Its activities include:

- Anti-cancer Activity.

- Immune-modulatory effect.

- Wound healing effects.

- Anti-nephro-toxicity effect.

- Hepato-protective activity.

- Anti-malarial activity.

- Anti-oxidant activity.

- Anti-fungal activity.

- Anti-bacterial activity.

- Anti-viral activity.

- Anti- inflammatory effect.

- Neuro-protective effective

- Anti-diabetic activity.

Neem modulates immune response via anti inflammatory mechanisms. It activates cells of adaptive immune system. It has been shown to be antiviral, antifungal, and antibacterial.

During inflammation, transcription factor NF-kB promotes the expression of inflammatory enzymes such as COX-2 and 5-LOX. Neem's active ingredient or compounds in the seed oil extract inhibit NF-kB thereby inhibiting expression of COX-2 and 5-LOX. Neem oil increased the production of IFN- gamma. Higher IFN-gamma increased the production of adaptive and innate immune cells, such as Th 1 cells and Cytotoxic T cells. Cytotoxic T cells directly kill the virus and mitigate the infection. They are effective against Polio virus and Herpes simplex virus type −1.

The antibacterial activity of Neem is seen with Neem bark extract and Neem seed oil extract. Dental plaque is sequential colonization of bacteria on the tooth surface. One gram of plaque contains nearly 100,000,000,000 bacteria. Neem bark and seed oil extracts exhibit antibacterial effect through inhibition of plaque formation and slowing their growth effectively. Neem seed oil has Azadiractin which disrupts the cell wall of bacteria and fungi. Cell wall disruption leads to leakage of intracellular content. Leakage of intracellular content leads to disturbance in osmotic pressure, the eventual death of bacteria or fungi.

**Recommended Dose in studies**

- Maintenance dose: 12 ml. of Neem oil

- For congestive heart failure: 250 mg/day Sodium nimbidinate (an active compound in Neem)

- For Anti ulcer effect: 60 - 120mg/day Neem bark extract

## (e) Garlic (Allium sativum)

Garlic is widely cultivate and use for culinary and medicinal purposes. Use of garlic dates back nearly 2700 BC years in ancient of Chinese, Sumerian, and Indian an Egyptian cultures. Medicinal effects of garlic attributed to its organic sulfur compounds. Garlic contains 105 chemical compounds include non-volatile compounds – Minerals, Vitamins, Saponins, Phenolic compounds; and volatile compounds - Organo-sulfur compounds. The minerals include Manganese, Zinc, Selenium, and Germanium. Vitamins include A, C, B1, B2, B3 and B6. Garlic also has Flavonoids including Rutin, Quercetin, Naringin, and Saponins like Eruboside-B, and Beta-chlorogenin. The volatile compounds include 33 organosulphur compounds which constitutes 2-3 % of fresh garlic.

The active organosulphur compounds of garlic are present in two classes: L- Cystein sulfoxides and Gamma-glutamyl-L-cysteine – peptides. Allin (S-Allyl-L-cysteine sulfoxide) is a major organosulphur compounds in garlic. Chopping, crushing, or chewing of garlic converts allin to allicin. Most of the medicinal benefits are derived from allicin and its metabolites such as: S-allylmercaptoglutathione (SAMG), S-allylmercaptocysteine (SAMC) and S-allyl-L-cysteine (SAC).

**Health Benefits of Garlic**

Garlic is shown to benefit the following health conditions

- Cardiovascular Health

  o Anti-hypertensive

  o Anti-atherosclerotic

  o Anti-thrombotic

- Cancer

    - Pro-apoptotic

    - Immune-therapeutic

- Antibiotic

    - Antibacterial

    - Antifungal

    - Anti-parasitic

    - Antiviral

- Immune-modulatory

- Anti-inflammatory

Garlic organo-sulphur compounds modulate immune cells and immune cell cytokines from innate as well as adaptive immune system through their anti-oxidative properties and anti-inflammatory properties. Garlic organo-sulphur compounds mitigate allergy. Garlic organo-sulphur compounds mitigate several diseases such as cardiovascular disease, obesity, gastric ulceration, and cancer through modulation of immune system.

Garlic organo-phosphorus compounds promote proliferation of innate immune cells including Natural Killer Cells, Gamma delta-T cells and Macrophages. Proliferation of innate immune cells leads to following activities of garlic: Anti – microbial, Anti – bacterial, Anti – viral, Anti – fungal.

Garlic compounds such as ajoene promotes activation of anti-inflammatory cytokine IL-10. IL-10 is needed for proliferation of anti-inflammatory Th2 cells. Th2 cells stimulate proliferation of antibody-producing B cells to produce IgA. IgA is an antibody that plays a crucial role in the immune function of mucus membranes.

Garlic inhibits enzymes such as ERK1/2 that are involved in inflammation signaling. Garlic inhibits transcription factor NF-kB which is responsible for transcription of inflammatory genes

Garlic mitigates allergy reaction by reducing production of histamines in basophils. Histamines are implicated in antigen-specific (e.g. nuts, shellfish, pollen) allergy response.

Garlic can modulate many systemic diseases including Gastric, Colorectal, and Pancreatic Cancer. Allicin from garlic induces apoptosis through JNK pathway activation and mitochondrial Bax translocation in cells. Aged garlic extract increased the cytotoxicity of T-cell lineage, which in turn targets the cancer cells. Garlic oil has been shown to lower ulceration by lowering oxidative stress and pro-inflammatory cytokines such as IL-10 and IL-12.

Garlic modulates the low-grade inflammation by reducing IL-6 and MCP-1.-2 in human pre-adipocytes in obese individuals. Garlic promotes anti-oxidant and anti-inflammatory environment thereby lowering atherosclerosis and hypertension.

**Recommended Dose in studies**

- Maintenance dose: 4gm of fresh garlic, 800mg dried garlic

- For Cardiovascular benefits: 1200-2400mg of aged garlic extract once a day.

- For Immune-modulation: 2,560 mg per day of aged garlic extract.

Onion is a complete functional food. It is widely cultivated and use for culinary and medical purposes. Onion's first documented medicinal use dates back 3,500 in the Egyptian Codex Ebers. Medicinal effects of Onion are attributed to Phenolic compounds, Minerals, Fiber, Organic sugar, and Organic sulfur compounds. Onion has non-volatile compounds which include minerals, vitamins, phenolic compounds, organic sugars, and fiber. It also has volatile compounds which are primarily organo-sulfur compounds. The minerals include Manganese, Zinc, Selenium, Potassium, and Phosphorus. The Vitamins include C, B1, B2, B3, B6, and E. Onion has 22 volatile organosulphur compounds of two classes: L-cysteine sulfoxides and Gamma-glutamyl-L-cysteine peptides. Allin (S-allyl-L-cysteine sulfoxide) is a major organosulphur compounds in onion. Chopping, crushing or chewing of onion converts alliin to allicin

Most of the medicinal benefits are derived from allicin and its metabolite such as:S-allylmercaptoglutathione (SAMG), S-allylmercaptocysteine (SAMC), and S-allyl-L-cysteine (SAC) similar to garlic

Onion is one of the richest sources of dietary phenolic compounds. Phenolic compounds exert their medicinal benefits through their anti-oxidant and anti-inflammatory properties. Quercetin and its derivatives represent 90% of the phenolic compounds in onion.

Health benefits of Onion include:

- Glucose control in diabetes

- Cardiovascular Health

    o Anti-hypertensive

- o Atherosclerotic

- • Anticancer

    - o Colorectal

    - o Laryngeal

    - o Oesophageal

    - o Gastric

    - o Prostrate

- • Immune health

    - o Anti-allergy

- • Antibiotic

    - o Anti-bacterial

    - o Anti-fungal

    - o Anti-parasitic

    - o Anti-viral

- • Anti-inflammatory

The organosulphur compounds in onion, selenium and quercetin promote proliferation of innate immune cells such as: Anti-infection CD16+ Natural Killer Cells. The proliferation of innate immune cell leads to Anti-microbial, anti-bacterial, anti-viral and anti-fungal effects.

Quercetin inhibits enzymes such as Lipoxygenase that are involved in inflammation signaling. Quercetin inhibits cytokines such as IL-6 and IL-8 that lea to inflammation. Onion inhibits transcription factor NF-kB which is responsible for transcription of inflammatory genes that cause "Cytokine Storm" such as: TNF-alpha, IL-1beta, IL-12, IL-6 and MCP-1.

Onion mitigates allergy reaction by reducing production of histamines in basophils. Histamines are implicated in antigen-specific (e.g. nuts, shellfish, pollen) allergy response.

**Recommended Dose in studies**

- Maintenance dose: 50 gm of fresh onion, 20 gm dried onion

- For Diabetes benefits: 100 gm of onion per day

- For Hypertension: 162 mg/day of quercetin from onion

- For Immune support: 250 – 500 mg/kg/day of onion extract

Ginger is one of the most commonly consumed dietary condiments in the world. Rhizome (roots) is the main portion of ginger that is consumed. Medical use of ginger dates back nearly 5,000 years in ancient of Chinese and Indian cultures. Medicinal effects of ginger attributed to its Gingerol compounds.

More than 100 chemical compounds have been identified so far in ginger. These include minerals, vitamins and Gingerols. Minerals include Calcium, Phosphorus, Manganese, Zinc, Iron, Copper, and Germanium. Vitamins include C. Ginger also has carotenoids. Gingerols has specific compounds with known medicinal benefits. They include [6]-Gingerol, [8]-Gingerol, [10]-Gingerol, [6]-shogaol

**Health benefits of Ginger**

The target of active compounds in ginger includes the following:

- Inhibition of VEGF

- Activation of G0/G1 phase

- Suppression of TNF & NF-kB

- Inhibition of IFN-gamma

- Inhibition of cycloxigenase

- Inhibition of Bcl2 & Survivin

- Inhibition of Interleukins

- Activation of P53

- Inhibition of Lypoxygenase

- Activation of Bax

Ginger has its effects by modifying the following components of metabolism

- Inflammatory Enzymes
    - Lypoxygenase
    - Cycloxygenase
- Inflammatory Cytokines
    - Interleukins
    - Interferon-gamma
    - TNF-alpha
- Transcription Factor
    - NF-kB
- Cell Growth Regulators
    - G0/G1 phase activators
- Cell Death Regulators
    - P53
    - Bcl2
    - Survivin
    - Bax
- Angiogenesis Regulators
    - VEGF

Ginger exhibits following biological effects:

- Anti-Bacterial activity

- Anti-diabetic

- Gastro protective effects

- Anti-obesity activity

- Hepato-protective activity

- Anti-tumor effect

- Immune System

- Neuro-protective Activity

- Inhibition of inflammatory activity

- Photo protection effect

Gingerols modulates the immune system through their anti-inflammatory properties. Ginger essential oil exhibit antimicrobial effects. Gingerols alleviates allergy symptoms through inhibition of histamine release. Gingerols relieve Asthma symptoms by inhibiting airway contraction.

Inflammation leads to harmful disproportionate immune response. Gingerol inhibits enzymes such as COX -2 an 5-LOX that are involved in inflammation signaling. Gingerol inhibits transcription factor NF-kB which is responsible for transcription of inflammatory genes that cause "cytokine storm" such as: TNF-alpha, IL-1beta, IL-8

Ginger essential oil has antibacterial and antifungal activities through cell membrane disruption.

Under asthmatic conditions Ca++ ions enter the airway smooth muscle (ASM) cells and cause contraction of airway. Extended contraction of airway worsens the asthmatic symptoms. Gingerol prevents Ca2+ ion entry by inhibiting the calcium channels on ASM cells. Gingerol inhibition of calcium channels leads to alleviation of asthma symptoms.

**Recommended Dose in studies**

- Maintenance dose: 250 mg to 4.8 gm/day

- For pain benefits: 2gm/day

- For sugar control: 1,600 mg/day

- For migraine: 250 mg in a single dose orally.

- Nausea: 250 mg to 2 gm/day

# CHAPTER 26

## Definitions and Key concepts

"Doctors are great-- as long as you don't need them" – Edward E. Rosenbaum

**1. What is a non-specific defense mechanism?**

Response is immediate and the same for all pathogens (Phagocytes and physical barriers).

**2. What is a specific defense mechanism?**

Response is slower and specific to each pathogen (T and B).

**3. Name an example of a physical barrier?**

Skin, epithelial cells covered in mucus, Hydrochloric acid.

**4. What is Phagocytosis?**

The mechanism by which phagocytes engulf particles (bacteria, viruses, fungi) to form phagosomes is called phagocytosis.

**5. What are Pathogens?**

The Micro-organisms that cause disease are called Pathogens.

**6. What is an Antigen?**

A molecule that triggers an immune response by lymphocytes (usually on the outer surface of a pathogen) is called an antigen.

## 7. What is a Lymphocyte?

A type of white blood cell responsible for the (specific) immune response becomes activated in the presence of an antigen. Two types: B and T.

## 8. What is Immunity?

The means by which the body protects itself from infection is called immunity.

## 9. What does Phagocyte (macrophage) do?

Engulf pathogens, where it is broken down by enzymes.

## 10. What is an Antibody?

A protein produced by lymphocytes in response to the presence of an antigen.

## 11. What is Vaccination?

The introduction of appropriate dead or disabled antigens by injection or by mouth to an individual is called vaccination.

## 12. What are Commensals?

The bacteria living on the skin that compete for nutrients and space with other pathogenic bacteria are called commensals.

## 13. What is an Inflammation?

It is caused by phagocytes at the site of infection, which contains dead pathogens and phagocytes (known as pus).

## 14. What is an Epidemic?

When a disease spreads between thousands of people in an area is called an epidemic..

## 15. What is a Pandemic?

When a disease spreads across the world is called a pandemic.

## 16. What is a B lymphocyte?

Develop from stem cells in bone marrow, lymphatic tissue, spleen, and lymph nodes.

## 17. What is a T lymphocyte?

Develop from stem cells in bone marrow and mature in the thymus

## 18. What do B lymphocytes do?

Humoral immunity- produce antibodies when activated – produce Memory cells that can be activated really quickly and produce antibodies straight away second time round.

## 19. What do T lymphocytes do?

Cell mediated immunity- Destroy cells that are, infected by virus, - cancerous,- transplanted cells. They recognize these cells as non-self because of antigens presented on their surface.

## 20. What types of T cells are there?

These are Memory cell, Helper cells, cytotoxic cells and Suppressor T cells.

## 21. What are Memory T cells?

They stay in the lymphatic system in readiness to respond quickly to a future infection.

## 22. What are Helper T cells?

They start immune response; activate B cells which produce antibodies that exact with the antigen. They can be infected by HIV.

## 23. What are leucocytes?

A type of white blood cells called leucocytes.

## 24. What are Cytotoxic T cells?

They kill the body's abnormal cells (as they show foreign antigens, like virus infected cells and cancer cells). Killing by destroying the cell membrane with perform (protein that inserts itself into the cell membrane and opens a pore).

## 25. What are suppressor T cells?

They produce chemical signals (cytokines) that suppress the activities of other T cells, helping to end the immune response.

## 26. What is Antigenic Variability?

Diseases such as influenza have 100s of different strains and, therefore, each one has different antigens.

## 27. What is the primary response?

The initial response to an antigen to produce antibodies in an individual is called primary response.

## 28. What is the secondary response?

When the infection is seen for a second time and is when a, delayed response is seen with a reduced amount of antigen. It's more rapid so that the pathogen can be destroyed before it fully infects the body and causes disease.

## 29. What is called when antibody binds to an antigen?

It is called an Antigen-antibody complex.

## 30. What does the antigen-antibody complex do?

It immobilizes the virus particles so they cannot latch onto cells, which makes it easier for phagocytes to track the antigens down.

## 31. What else do antigens cause?

Agglutination, stimulation of phagocytes, precipitation, prevention of attachment to cell

## 32. What is agglutination?

Antibodies stick to the antigens on the surface of the pathogen and can stick to many at a time immobilizing them and allowing macrophages to engulf them easier.

## 33. What are monoclonal antibodies?

Many of the same type of antibody formed from one type of plasma B lymphocyte.

## 34. When are monoclonal antibodies used?

In immune-assay (pregnancy tests, doping tests for athletes), cancer treatments, transplant surgery.

## 35. How can monoclonal antibodies be used in cancer treatments?

The monoclonal antibody can be made to attach themselves to cancer cells, and also be able to activate a cytotoxic drug (one that kills cells). Therefore, the drug will be activated by the cells to which monoclonal antibodies are attached, thus killing the cancer cells and leaving other cells relatively unharmed.

## 36. How can monoclonal antibodies be used in transplant surgery?

Even with close matching of organs, a transplanted organ will normally suffer some sort of rejection because of the action of T cells. Monoclonal antibodies can be used to "knock out" these specific T cells.

## 37. What is Immunization?

It is a creating artificial immunity by vaccination.

## 38. What is Vaccination?

Acquiring immunity to a disease using a vaccine or special antigenic material to stimulate the formation of appropriate antibodies is called vaccination.

## 39. What is vaccine?

It is a preparation of antigenic material that stimulates antibody production (primary response) and gives active immunity against the disease

## 40. What are the four different ways of immunity?

Naturally acquired immunity, artificially acquired immunity, naturally acquired passive immunity, artificial acquired passive immunity.

## 41. What are the types of vaccines?

-Live pathogens (attenuated/weakened e.g. Rubella)

-Killed virulent micro-organism, e.g. Whooping cough, influenza

-Isolated antigens, e.g. influenza

-Genetically engineered antigens, e.g. Hepatitis B

-Modified toxins, e.g. Diphtheria


## 42. What is herd immunity?

Vaccinations protect not only those who have been vaccinated, but also those who have not. It reduces the pathogen in the population so it's not transmitted from person to person.

## 43. What is the problem with oral vaccinations?

They are proteins, which are digested by enzymes of the G.I.tract.

# CHAPTER 27

# What we should know about COVID-19

"It is reasonable to expect the doctor to recognize that science may not have all the answers to problems of health and healing." – Norman Cousins-

COVID 19 is the name of the virus implicated in the 2020-21 global pandemic. We must know how it works and how it affects people leading to fatal outcomes in many cases. Like other viruses, it is a form of Corona virus which has been infecting humans for centuries. And like all other viruses it is also an opportunistic virus, which causes serious symptoms in those individuals who have some co-morbidity or those who have their immunity is compromised in one way or the other. The healthy people who have their immunity in perfect health may not even know the infection in their body or a minimally affected symptom with them. It is inappropriate to just blame this virus for all the adverse outcomes during this pandemic. We as individuals and the government are partially to blame for ignoring the root cause for the death and disability during this pandemic.

Not many individuals pay attention to strengthening the general immunity of our population. By supporting blanket capitalism and commercialization, we have allowed sale of liquor, cigarettes and tobacco, and other packaged and chemical-laden foods freely to the public. We have not taken steps to remove adulteration of our food with toxic chemicals. There are no intensive government programs guiding individuals towards preventive health. Hospitals and medicines are considered as the ultimate cure. Food is not treated as medicine. This is one of the reasons that the virus has created so much havoc in the world. Our lifestyle choices have deteriorated our immunity.

We must know how our army of protective cells in the body, acts to protect us from this virus. We have macrophages, which affects IL-1 beta, IL-6, and IL-18.

- Dendritic cells affect TNF-Alpha. T cells affect IFN-gamma, TNF-alpha, IL-6 and IL-18. Fibroblasts affect IL-6 and IL-18, Endothelium also affects IL-1 beta.

- The clinical features of these cytokines appear in the body as fever with IFN-gamma, TNF-alpha, IL- 1 Beta, and IL-6.

- An impaired hematopoietic function is produced by IFN-gamma and TNF-alpha.

- Debilitating state of the body and hyperlipidemia is also produced by TNF-alpha.

- The Liver is damaged with TNF-alpha and IL-18.

- Acute kidney injury and anemia are produced by IL-6.

- Acute phase proteins are seen with IL-1 beta and IL-6.

In a normal individual who has proper immunity when the virus attacks the body, the cells produce a cytokine IL-1 alpha which alerts the army of Neutrophils, NK cells and Monocytes and these kill the virus at the spot. If the virus reaches the macrophages, they are the second line of defense to kill the virus. When the virus enters the blood, the pDC cells (plasmacytoid Dendritic Cells) alert the T cells and start producing antibodies IgM and IgG to tackle the virus through alerting the B cells. In this way, the problem is tackled without any damage to the body, naturally, through multiple layers of defense.

In an individual with compromised immunity when the virus attacks, his or her macrophages do not kill the virus and production of IFN-alpha from the cells is also delayed so the Neutrophils, Monocytes and NK cells do not receive any message to activate. The infected cells through the ACE2R receptors produce Bradykinin, which increases the vascular permeability. The infected cells also presents to the cDC (conventional Dendritic Cells) and which in turn affect the Th1 cells. These Th1 cells affect to release IL-8 and cause neutrophil migration and produce inflammation. Th1 also release TNF-alpha and through Phospholipase 2 cause inflammation. Th1 also release IL-6, which increases fibrinogen, and leakage of coagulation factors and the formation of micro thrombi. Macrophages on the other hand through the NLRP3 pathway release IL-18 cytokine, which also fuels the furry of already existing Inflammation. This pathway also releases another cytokine IL-1 beta, responsible for hyper-ferritinemia and fever, and also contributes to inflammation and tissue damage by increasing the Glucuronidases.


THE END